HEALTHY
TRAVELER$_x$

THE HEALTHY TRAVELER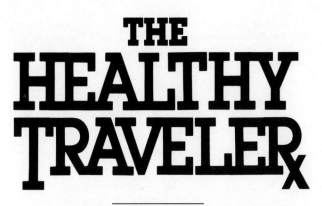

AN INDISPENSABLE GUIDE TO STAYING HEALTHY AWAY FROM HOME

BETH WEINHOUSE

Foreword by Kenneth R. Dardick, M.D.

PUBLISHED BY POCKET BOOKS NEW YORK

Another *Original* publication of POCKET BOOKS

POCKET BOOKS, a division of Simon & Schuster, Inc.
1230 Avenue of the Americas, New York, N.Y. 10020

ISBN: 0-671-61445-2

First Pocket Books trade paperback printing February, 1987

10 9 8 7 6 5 4 3 2 1

POCKET and colophon are registered trademarks
of Simon & Schuster, Inc.

Printed in the U.S.A.

To my parents, with love

ACKNOWLEDGMENTS

My thanks to the many physicians, researchers, and others who took the time to speak with me and provide information, and especially to the following: the fine staffs of the National Institutes of Health and the Centers for Disease Control, Dr. Vincenzo Marcolongo of the International Association for Medical Assistance to Travelers, and Dr. Kenneth Dardick of Immunization Alert.

My appreciation also to James Ryan, for his superb technical suport, and to his wife and my friend Nina Berler for her equally valuable emotional support. I am also grateful to Matthew Mosner, Lisa Weiler, and John Steidl for their foreign language translations. And I could not have written this book without the following people: my family and my good friend Beth Sobel, who have been my principal traveling companions; Rachel Hager, my expert fact-checker; Jan Goodwin, who commiserated with me during the "writing process"; Pam Dorman, my editor, who guided me through each step; and Stuart Krichevsky, my agent, who encouraged me to pursue this project from the beginning.

CONTENTS

Foreword

A few years ago one of my patients who teaches at the University of Connecticut came to me with this request: "I'm going on sabbatical for a year and will be visiting about ten countries in Asia and the Pacific. What shots will I need?" After a difficult hour of research that included searching reference books, making numerous telephone calls to the health department, and consulting experts at the Centers for Disease Control, I emerged with some tentative recommendations for my patient. He and I then spent another hour or so discussing his specific travel plans and agreed upon what preventive measures he would need for this trip.

On that day I decided there had to be a better way to advise my patients who were traveling. But it's no simple job to keep track of over two hundred countries throughout the world. Health situations are constantly changing. New diseases such as Lyme disease, AIDS, and resistant strains of malaria appear with some frequency.

This was the beginning of my serious interest in the field now known as travel medicine. It led to the development of the Immunization Alert℗ international health database, a computerized system that keeps track of health conditions in over two hundred countries and helps physicians and health officials give accurate advice to their traveling patients.

Encounters like the one I described above occur daily as travelers seek advice about staying healthy while traveling. But they don't always receive the proper advice, for several reasons.

First, not all doctors are interested in advising travelers. They may either refer their patients to another source of information, such as the local health department, or—sad to say—they may try to help and in so doing rely on outdated or inaccurate information. Recently some researchers in Canada discovered that over one third of doctors they surveyed were using references for travel advice that were over five years old! This just isn't acceptable when you consider that there may be as many as fifty changes each year in the official recommendations for travel abroad.

Some travelers simply focus on the limited question, "What shots will I need?" rather than asking the broader question, "What health precautions should I consider for this trip?" The first question only deals with the legal requirements to cross international borders. The second question recognizes that there are many health issues beyond "shots" for the traveler to consider. Jet lag, motion sickness, traveler's diarrhea, altitude sickness, and auto accidents are all examples of the broader issues travelers need to address before they leave.

Other travelers ask about health precautions, but fail to realize that the answers will depend on many factors—including their own medical history, medications they take, where they will travel within the country, how long and during what seasons they will stay there, even their own travel experience and knowledge. My patients often call me on the telephone to ask advice for their upcoming trip. I always tell them that the answer is too complex to squeeze into a two-minute phone call and invite them to come in to discuss their *own* situation in detail.

Beth Weinhouse discusses and answers these questions and many others in her book. She is a veteran world traveler. Her own experiences and her skill as a journalist are brought together to create a useful reference for both the novice and the professional traveler.

The Healthy Traveler is an encyclopedic reference of health issues for *all* travelers. This book guides you through all the preparations necessary before you leave, tells you what to pack, how to deal with common problems, and how to prepare for unique concerns like pregnancy, travel with children, travel by the disabled, and travel by the elderly. There are sections with lots of practical advice about diet and exercise while traveling. There are wonderful hints on relaxing fatigued feet and aching muscles by applying alternating hot and cold washcloths (it sounds inviting just reading about it!). There is even a section on the proper care of contact lenses while traveling.

Read this book as soon as you start planning your trip. The general information will apply wherever you travel. The sections on jet lag, diet, motion sickness, and health insurance are especially important before the trip begins.

Then, when you have a specific trip in mind, read closely those sections that apply to your itinerary. At the same time make an appointment with your own family doctor or a specialist in travel medicine. Discuss your specific plans, including the level of hygiene expected in your destination and the length of your stay. If you will be spending more than a few weeks away you should probably obtain prescriptions for medications such as antibiotics or medication for motion sickness and traveler's diarrhea. Have your doctor explain in detail when they should (or should not) be used. This will be especially helpful if you will be in an isolated area with no medical care at hand.

And don't forget to take this book with you while traveling. It will be an invaluable reference on such topics as first aid, sports injuries, dealing with emergencies like a hotel fire or earthquake, and obtaining drugs in a foreign country. Beth Weinhouse has provided a marvelous service for the traveler by collecting so much important information in one place.

There is no question that traveling is not the same as staying home. But that's why you're traveling! The message I give my patients, and the message in this book, is to enjoy your trip; but first spend a little time and effort learning about the places you will visit and what precautions will help you stay healthy . . .

. . . and send me a postcard!

Kenneth R. Dardick, M.D.
Center for International Health
Storrs, CT

SEPTEMBER 1986

Introduction

Nothing can ruin a much-anticipated vacation or an important business trip like a health problem. Yet according to the National Institutes of Health, one in three Americans will become ill abroad. And these illnesses range from mild cases of flu and "Montezuma's Revenge" to more serious sicknesses such as malaria and yellow fever. With thirty million Americans traveling out of the country every year, that's a lot of medical problems. Add to these figures the countless numbers who endure minor annoyances like jet lag, motion sickness, blisters, bug bites, and sunburn, and you realize that an awful lot of people are suffering while they're away from home.

As an experienced traveler and a medical writer, I always assumed I was immune to these problems. Yet when I recall most of my voyages, no matter how enjoyable they were, I can also usually remember some health problem I encountered. For a normally healthy person, my international medical history is pretty dismal: I've suffered from motion sickness on the Aegean Sea, and been tortured by the high altitude of the Peruvian Andes and the heat of the Israeli desert. I managed to get fleas and eat poisonous mushrooms in such a civilized place as France. Even my seemingly innocuous "fun in the sun" vacations held their perils: I stepped on a sea urchin in Barbados, was stung by a jellyfish in St. Maarten, got badly sunburned in St. Croix, contracted a terrible cold in Mexico, and came down with a case of "turista" in Jamaica. And almost everywhere I've been I've had to deal with jet lag, strange food, and exhaustion. Horror stories I've heard from friends have been even worse: food poisoning, amoebic dysentery, broken legs, emergency surgery . . . the list goes on and on.

But it's no wonder travelers suffer. Suddenly, they're confronted with unfamiliar food, more physical activity than usual, time differences, and a completely new environment (whether it be a cruise ship, mountaintop, island beach, or Amazon jungle). They may be walking more, eating more, sleeping less. And instead of the friendly germs they've met at home and to which they've built up immunity, they're confronted with completely unfamiliar organisms that throw their bodies for a loop.

Once travelers fall ill, they're less capable of dealing with the situation than they would be at home. Consider the case of a couple flying down to Rio for Carnival. After a night of partying they are left with uncomfortable stomachaches and hangovers, but they didn't bring any medication from home—they were trying to keep their luggage light. The Brazilian pharmacy is full of unfamiliar bottles with Portuguese labels. What should they do?

Or a businessman must make an important presentation in Tokyo when he comes down with a runny nose, sneezes, general achiness, and fatigue. If he doesn't get rid of his cold fast, he'll never be able to concentrate on his business meeting. What began as just an annoying, garden-variety cold could ruin the entire trip—and crucial business to boot.

But there's no reason for vacationers to lie in their hotel beds while the sun shines outside, or executives to sniffle through business meetings, because most ailments that afflict travelers are completely preventable. After all, you protect yourself automatically at home: by adjusting your diet in order to feel well, wearing the right clothes for the weather, and making sure that you get enough sleep. There's no reason why, with a minimum of planning, good health away from home can't be just as automatic.

The biggest reason for health neglect is ignorance. Americans are accustomed to safe water, food, and swimming areas, and they regard cuts, scrapes, and mosquito bites as mere nuisances. But once anyone leaves his "home turf," these assumptions are dangerous. Cuts and blisters can easily get infected. Mosquito bites can carry malaria, encephalitis, and yellow fever.

Destination travel guides usually address the subject of health perfunctorily—perhaps advising people to check on immunizations, or to avoid the water in certain areas. But this general advice doesn't begin to give travelers the knowledge you need to protect yourself from health hazards . . . and the statistics show the results. The information omitted from these books can be crucial: For example, most people know that drinking contaminated water can bring on a case of "Montezuma's Revenge," but how many people know that swimming in some water (especially with an open cut or an ear infection) can also bring on travelers' diarrhea? Obviously not many, since an estimated one-third to one-half of all travelers to Mexico succumb to turista. But what good is avoiding the water anyway, if you arrive at your destination so dehydrated and jet lagged from the plane ride that it will be days before you feel like yourself? If the journey is only a week long, or less, you'll be going home before you're back to normal.

Many people avoid travel health planning because they mistakenly believe it takes too much time, and detracts from the hedonism of a much-anticipated vacation, or the crucial planning of an important business trip. They're wrong.

Planning for good health while traveling should be as automatic as maintaining good health at home. There's no need for anyone to become a paranoid hypochondriac in order to avoid illness abroad. Once the basics are mastered, they become as routine a part of preparing for a voyage as packing a toothbrush.

The best way to use this book is first to read it through *before* you plan a trip, so that you have time to go from cover to cover and familiarize yourself with all the health issues involved in traveling. Then, when you're ready to make those reservations for Paris, check out the contents and read all the chapters that seem applicable to your voyage. Finally, take this book along with you, so that you can refer to it for help and advice as your trip progresses.

Whether you're traveling for business or pleasure, you have only limited time to accomplish your goals—whether these goals are sales, contracts, relaxation, or adventure. Good health is essential to having a successful, happy trip.

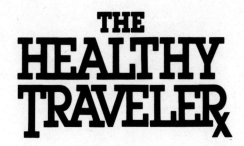

1 | Making Your Reservations . . . for a Healthy Trip

Health planning is the key to a carefree vacation, and should be part of every pre-vacation itinerary. When you make your plane reservations, also arrange with your doctor for any needed immunizations. When you decide what clothes to bring, also pack a light, travelers' medical kit. When you research the culture and history of your destination, also make sure to check on the climate, food, water, and endemic diseases. Do the work before you go, and put the odds in your favor for a healthy trip.

What to Bring

A first-aid kit is crucial for any vacation or business trip, no matter where you're going or for how long. By deciding in advance what you need, and by taking the time to shop around for compact tubes and bottles (many common toiletries and medications now come in special travel sizes), you can make sure that your kit is small and light (and won't take up room in your suitcase you'd rather use for that extra pair of shoes).

The best way to decide what to bring is to assemble a basic kit, and then personalize it according to your needs and destination. Obviously, a young couple traveling to London won't need the same supplies as a family with small children going trekking in Nepal.

A good basic kit should include:

- A multi-purpose antibiotic, such as tetracycline
- Aspirin or a recommended substitute, such as acetaminophen or ibuprofen

- Cold and cough remedies, such as an over-the-counter decongestant and antihistamine
- Diarrhea medication
- A mild laxative
- An antacid
- A sunscreen
- Insect repellent
- Antifungal and anti-itch agents
- An antibacterial cream or spray
- An Ace™ bandage
- Adhesive tape and gauze
- Band-Aids™, cotton swabs, and tissues
- Alcohol wipes or rubbing alcohol
- Scissors and tweezers
- A thermometer
- A first aid manual (you should be able to find a paperback version in most bookstores)

Make sure all items are clearly marked, and include the expiration date on medications that deteriorate with age (even common medications like aspirin deteriorate over time). Pack the kit in a container with a waterproof cover, and keep it with your hand luggage for easy access. (Avoid bringing any aerosol sprays if you're flying, since pressure changes can cause them to explode.) Remember, you don't need massive quantities of each item listed, just enough to tide you over in case something unexpected occurs or until you can get more. Not only will you save money by bringing this small medical kit along (because similar supplies are often quite costly if purchased abroad or at a tourist resort), you'll be sure of having what you need when you need it.

The contents listed above should take care of most of the minor problems you may encounter away from home, but you may want to modify or add to this basic kit depending on your itinerary. Think through your destinations and planned activities. Will you be camping? Perhaps you should bring along extra medication in case of bug bites or poison ivy. And depending on where you're camping, you might want to bring along a snakebite kit, too. Will you be skiing, hiking, or playing other sports in which you don't normally participate all year long? Maybe it's a good idea to take along some ointment to soothe sore muscles, and a few extra bandages. Do you suffer from allergies? Throw in another bottle of antihistamines or a decongestant just in case, since it's hard to know whether you'll be allergic to the plants, pollens, or foods in a strange destination. If you're allergic to insect bites and stings, be sure to take along a kit containing injectable epinephrine, in case of a severe allergic reaction.

Going on a cruise? Bring some anti–motion sickness medication, especially if you've never sailed before and don't know what to expect. Campers, backpackers, and people traveling to countries where the water isn't safe should bring water purification tablets, bleach, iodine, or an electric immersion coil and converter for boiling water (see chapter 4).

Some physicians recommend bringing along the drug diphenhydramine, as close to an all-purpose medication for travelers as there is. An antihistamine, diphenhydramine will relieve allergy symptoms, mild motion sickness, and even insomnia. Diphenhydramine is sold over-the-counter under the brand name Benadryl.

If you have children along, your medical kit should contain some special things just for them—for instance, liquid medications instead of pills. And all medications should have childproof caps. (Consult chapter 10—"Traveling with Children"—for specifics.)

Make sure you personalize your medical kit, too. If you're prone to hemorrhoids, vaginal infections, sinus problems or ear infections, for example—all common complaints—be sure to include whatever medication you usually find most effective. If you suffer from asthma, take along an extra inhaler. It may not be available away from home.

And your first aid kit should contain more than just "things"; it should contain information. Prepare a sheet of paper listing the immunization histories and pertinent medical information (chronic illnesses, prescription medications) of all travelers. Make sure to list medicines by the generic name as well as the brand name, so that foreign physicians and pharmacists can help provide you with the correct equivalent if necessary. (Generic names are more universal than brand names. Your doctor or pharmacist can help you identify generic names of common medications.) If possible, bring along a copy of your prescriptions, even though they may not be honored out of state, let alone out of the country. Also include a copy of prescriptions for eyeglasses or contact lenses, in case they are broken or lost while you are away. Always carry your physician's address and phone number with you in case you need to reach him or her while you're away.

Having your immunization history along can be very reassuring when traveling. If there's an outbreak of polio in an area you're visiting, you can be certain you're protected. If you step on a rusty nail, you'll know instantly when you received your last tetanus shot.

And make sure to include your health insurance identification card, too, along with a claim form. If you must seek medical attention without the proper papers, you may find yourself with reimbursement problems later.

Pills and Potions

Millions of Americans take prescription medication daily, and obviously, the medicines must travel with them. The best way to carry medication is in hand luggage, in case checked baggage is lost or stolen. As mentioned above, you should keep a copy of your prescription handy, for several reasons: 1) If you must replace your medication, the prescription, with the generic name listed as well as the brand name, and the strength and dosage, will make the job much easier, and 2) Customs officials may occasionally question mysterious-looking pill bottles. Having the prescription handy will speed your passage. Keeping medications in their original containers will also discourage unnecessary attention from customs agents.

It's also a good idea to take along a letter from your physician, including his address and phone number, describing your medical problems and treatment. (Diabetics who carry disposable syringes with them will find having a letter from their doctor especially helpful to ease the suspicions of customs officials.) Having this information will help both with customs and in case of medical emergencies later. Also ask your doctor to write out for you the generic name of your medication, as well as the trade names in the countries you will visit. The information is included in *The Merck Index,* 10th Ed. (1983), and also in *Martindale: The Extra Pharmacopoeia,* 28th Ed. (London: The Pharmaceutical Press, 1982). These books should be available in the public library's reference section. If not, ask a local hospital or university whether you can use their library.

One way of being sure not to run out of medication away from home is to calculate how much medicine you will need for the entire time you're away, then pack twice as much as you'll need. You may have to call your physician or pharmacist for extra medicine before you leave. If you're flying, pack half the medication in your carry-on baggage and the extra half in the baggage you check on the flight. Keep in mind, however, that if you are going to be away from home for more than a couple of weeks, it may *not* be a good idea to carry double your medication. Customs officials will be suspicious of drugs they consider to be in larger than "reasonable quantities," so if you pack a pharmacy's worth, you're likely to be stopped. For long trips, take just a bit more than you'll need—if you require refills while traveling, see chapter 12 for advice.

If you've ever wondered whether or not to leave the wad of cotton in your pill bottles after you've opened them, the answer is: Usually, no, but when traveling, yes. The cotton is not in the bottle to keep the pills fresh. (In fact, it can sometimes be contaminated with microorganisms.) The cotton is placed in the bottle at the factory to keep the pills from rattling around and breaking when being carried or shipped. So while you should leave the cotton out of your pill bottles at home, it's a good idea to put some cotton back into the bottles when you cart medication along on a trip. Taking plastic bottles rather than glass, and tablets or capsules rather than liquid medication, will also make traveling easier.

Another consideration when traveling with medication is whether or not conditions such as altered temperature (of the airplane's baggage hold or the tropical sun, for example) will affect the medication's potency. The answer depends on the specific medicine, but in general medications should be kept away from bright light, in a cool (not cold), dry place. Most medications should be kept away from direct sunlight, and away from wetness or humidity. Your physician should tell you if your medications have different storage requirements.

Vaccines, Immunizations, and Other Prudent Precautions

Preparing for a healthy trip starts with being healthy before you leave (although specific traveling tips for people with existing health problems are discussed in chapter 11). It's a good idea to have a thorough medical and dental checkup before you travel. Obviously, it's a lot better for your dentist to find a loose filling and fix it before you fly to Italy, than to have the filling fall out as you bite into some luscious Roman pizza. Make your doctor's appointment well in advance of your departure date, since some vaccinations must be given several weeks (and a few, even months) ahead of time to be effective. At the time of your examination, you can also ask your doctor for advice about preventing any specific health problems—allergies, asthma, hemorrhoids, vaginal infections, whatever—you are prone to.

Once you are away from home, even minor problems can take on major significance. For instance, most people take insect bites for granted, but there are plenty of places where a simple bug bite can lead to any number of serious diseases, including malaria, encephalitis, plague, or yellow fever. Or, though you may not have had a cold or virus in years, you can contract one shortly after arriving in a foreign locale.

That's because many health rules change when the setting does. Colds are a good example. Scientists have identified about one hundred variations of the virus that causes colds. Each time you get a cold, you build up immunity to that specific virus, but if you're exposed to a different one, you'll get sick again.

After you've lived in one place for several years, you've probably built up a natural immunity to many of the local bugs. But as soon as you travel any distance, your body will be exposed to unfamiliar viruses and you may very well get a cold . . . if not something worse. For this reason, American health officials are reporting a high incidence of flu-like upper respiratory infections among Americans returning from China.

But you don't have to accept sneezes and sniffles as the inevitable price you pay for traveling. Scientists now know that colds are not just spread by sneezing, sharing drinking glasses, or even kissing. Colds are frequently caused by hand-to-mouth, hand-to-nose, or hand-to-eye contact. For instance, if you shake hands with someone who has a cold, or you even ride a bus holding on to a strap that someone with a cold has just used, and then bite your nails or eat a sandwich, you could be infecting yourself with cold germs. So, one of the best ways to prevent colds is also the simplest: Reduce stress, get plenty of sleep, eat well . . . and wash your hands frequently. By keeping your hands clean, you are blocking one important route of disease transmission.

If colds were all travelers had to worry about, this book would hardly be necessary. Unfortunately, there are a host of exotic and unfamiliar diseases all over the world, and the traveler who intends to stay healthy had better be prepared.

When you visit your doctor for your pre-travel checkup, ask him if your routine vaccinations and immunizations are up to date. You should be immune to polio, measles, rubella (German measles), and mumps. You should also have had a tetanus and diphtheria booster within the last ten years.

After you've made sure these "regular" vaccinations are in order, ask your physician about any additional vaccines for your destination. But—and this is important—don't necessarily rely on your physician alone for advice, especially if you're traveling somewhere exotic. Many doctors are unfamiliar with immunization requirements, for the simple reason that they do not have much call for being expert. After all, how many times does a small-town doctor get asked what vaccines are required for a trip to Mozambique? And even if a physician tries to keep informed, it would be difficult for him to know every health problem affecting every country. Would most doctors have known, for example, about a recent mumps epidemic in Belgium, or a meningitis outbreak in Nepal? Call your doctor and ask him if he advises travelers, or has a special interest in the subject. If not, call a local university medical school's infectious disease department for help in finding a doctor with an interest in travelers' health, or a special travelers' health clinic.

The following are some general guidelines for immunization and protection against "travelers' diseases." For specific disease and immunization advice about your travel destination, see this chapter's section on information sources, chapter 13, listing travelers' health clinics across the country, and chapter 14—"Health Guide to the World."

Immunization for travelers can be divided into three categories: Recommended, optional, and legislated.

RECOMMENDED VACCINATIONS

Most Americans traveling to other parts of the world will not need any immunizations in addition to those they should have already received from their regular physicians (see above). Again, it is impossible to stress enough the importance of making sure that these vaccinations are up to date. All travelers should be protected against measles, mumps, rubella, tetanus, diphtheria, and polio. People traveling to developing countries should ask their physician about the advisability of a polio booster for extra insurance. In addition, people considered at special risk should ask their physicians if other vaccinations—such as the influenza or pneumococcal vaccine—would be helpful. (See chapter 11 for more advice for people with existing health problems and the elderly.) If you're headed to a country in the midst of a flu epidemic—and even the most developed nations have flu outbreaks—ask your doctor about amantadine (Symmetrel), a drug which can be taken temporarily, in place of a vaccine, to prevent the flu. In general, travelers to Canada, Europe, Australia, and New Zealand need not be unduly concerned about disease.

OPTIONAL VACCINATIONS

There are now ways to protect against such infectious diseases as hepatitis, meningococcal meningitis, typhoid, plague, and rabies. Travelers should take their own health into consideration, as well as their destination and the nature of their travel, when deciding upon pre-trip immunization. People who will be spending all of their time in large resorts and Western-style hotels, for example, will probably not need special immunizations. More adventurous travelers, who plan on exploring the countryside, jungles, or deserts of underdeveloped countries with poor hygiene and sanitation, should take precautions to prevent illness.

Hepatitis—Protection is available against both hepatitis A (infectious hepatitis) and hepatitis B (serum hepatitis). Immune serum globulin may be given to travelers voyaging to places where hepatitis A is prevalent. Those at risk include visitors spending three or more weeks in a developing country where they will be eating home-cooked meals or staying in facilities with poor sanitary conditions. Hepatitis A can be spread through food, especially shellfish. Voyagers to the Mediterranean area should be particularly careful of eating local shellfish.

To protect against hepatitis B, travelers at risk—usually those who will be having sexual contact with persons who may be infected—may be vaccinated (the vaccine is a series of three shots which must be given at least six months before a trip to provide protection), or more likely will receive hepatitis B immune globulin. Immune globulin is also given after suspected exposure to the virus, to help prevent the disease from developing.

Meningococcal meningitis—Meningitis occurs throughout the world, but often in epidemics (for example, recent epidemics occurred in India and Nepal). The vaccine is recommended for travelers planning to visit (especially for three weeks or longer) areas of a country experiencing an epidemic of this disease. The so-called "meningitis belt" is in sub-Saharan Africa, and includes such countries as Mauritania, Mali, Niger, Chad, Sudan, Ethiopia, and Somalia.

Typhoid fever—The risk of travelers getting typhoid fever is considered small, but there are areas of Africa, Asia, and Central and South America where food and water may be contaminated. Typhoid is one of the many travelers' diseases that can cause diarrhea. Other symptoms include chronic fever, skin rash, headache, and abdominal discomfort. Travelers to these areas should consider typhoid vaccine, since completely avoiding contaminated food and water is difficult. Some people prefer to take their chances, however, since the vaccine is not considered very effective, and it often causes unpleasant side effects such as pain at the site of the injection, fever, nausea, and headache. Even after receiving the vaccine, it's important for travelers to eat and drink carefully—only cooked foods or those that can be peeled, and only bottled, boiled, or purified water (see chapter 3 for more detailed information). An oral vaccine for typhoid, manufactured in Switzerland, is not yet available in the U.S.

Plague—Plague is spread to humans by rodents and fleas. While there are a few cases in the United States each year, countries that continue to report occasional outbreaks include parts of Africa, Asia, and South America. In most of these countries, the risk to travelers is limited to rural and semirural areas. Travelers to areas reporting an epidemic or outbreak of plague should consider receiving the plague vaccine (particularly if they do not plan to stay in urban areas with tourist accommodations), although the vaccine is now rarely considered necessary.

Rabies—Most travelers will not require rabies vaccinations, but those who might be at risk—including children visiting countries where rabies is prevalent—should consider immunization. All travelers should avoid contact with animals, even pets, unless they are certain the animal has been vaccinated against rabies. It's not necessary to be bitten to contract the disease; even a lick on skin with a small cut can transmit rabies. (It's important to know that the vaccine does not eliminate the need for treatment after exposure to the disease.)

Encephalitis—A virus that infects and inflames the brain cells, encephalitis may be passed along by mosquitoes or other insects. Again, it is most prevalent in underdeveloped parts of the world, and in areas where insect infestation has not been controlled. A vaccine against Japanese B encephalitis, which is prevalent in Asia, has been developed in Japan, although as of this writing it is considered experimental in the United States, and can only be obtained at about fifty centers in this country. Have your physician contact the Centers for Disease Control for more information if you are traveling to India, Bangladesh, eastern U.S.S.R., China, Korea, Nepal, Burma, Viet Nam, or northern Thailand. Travelers are considered at risk if they will be spending their time in rural areas, and will be away for at least several weeks.

LEGISLATED VACCINATIONS

Travelers to and from certain areas may be required to prove vaccination against cholera or yellow fever in order to be allowed entry into some countries. High-risk areas for these diseases can change from year to year or month to month, so travelers should check with their state or local health departments (which receive updated material from the Centers for Disease Control every two weeks) for current information.

Cholera is an intestinal infection which is rare in developed countries, but still prevalent in Africa, Asia, and the Middle East. The disease, which causes diarrhea, is spread through contaminated food and water. Cholera vaccine is not routinely recommended because it is not considered very effective, but some countries require an International Certificate of Vaccination against cholera as a condition for entry. You can get the blank certificate (to be completed by the physician giving the vaccination) from most city, county, and state health departments, as well as many private clinics and doctors' offices. Or you can send $2 to: Superintendent of Documents, U.S. Government Printing Office, Washington, D.C. 20402. Write the code 017-001-004405 on the envelope.

The vaccine is good for six months.

Check carefully: Some countries will not require a certificate if you are arriving from the U.S., but will if you are arriving from parts of Asia or Africa. If your itinerary includes several stops, make sure that you are prepared for each arrival. It's far better to receive the injection in the U.S. than at a foreign airport where you can't be certain of the sanitation. Also, if you arrive in a country without the proper immunization papers, you may be held in quarantine.

Even vaccinated persons should be careful about food and water in places where cholera is present—the vaccine is only considered about fifty percent effective against the disease. A recent cholera outbreak in Pakistan was traced to melons that had been injected with sugared water. In some developing countries, crops are fertilized with "midnight soil," which is human manure—a potent disease spreader. And contaminated raw fruits and vegetables are also responsible for many cases of cholera.

Yellow fever—Cases of yellow fever are usually reported from Africa and South America, but occasionally from Central America and the Caribbean as well. The disease is transmitted primarily by mosquitoes. People traveling to areas where yellow fever is reported should check with their state or local health departments, since the vaccine can only be administered at an approved Yellow Fever Vaccination Center. With the vaccine, travelers will receive an International Certificate of Vaccination, which is valid for ten years.

Smallpox—In May 1980 the World Health Organization declared the world to be free of smallpox. A smallpox vaccination certificate is no longer required by any country as a condition of entry for international travelers. Since May 1983, smallpox vaccine is no longer distributed for civilian use in the U.S.

Before receiving *any* vaccination, make sure your physician knows your health status, whether you have any chronic conditions, what medications you are taking, whether or not you are pregnant, and if you have any allergies (especially to eggs).

Vaccinations are not available for all, or even most, of the diseases that travelers run the risk of contracting. Gastrointestinal diseases, for instance, are the most common diseases for travelers. These diseases are usually caused by viruses, parasites, or bacteria. So far, there are no vaccines to protect against these diseases, but travelers can protect themselves by exercising caution about food and drink, and practicing proper hygiene. Specifics for avoiding gastrointestinal illnesses—and treating them if they occur—will be discussed in chapter 3.

Malaria and Other Insect-Borne Diseases

Besides taking precautions against contaminated food and water, it is crucial that travelers protect themselves against insect-borne diseases, especially malaria. Malaria is one of the most common infectious diseases in the world today, and one of the biggest health risks to travelers, but as yet there is no vaccine to protect against it. Spread by mosquitoes, malaria is present in much of the world, including Asia, Africa, Central and South America, and the Middle East. A quick way to remember countries where malaria is present: The disease tends to favor warm climates, and countries near the equator (45° N latitude to 45° S latitude), such as East Africa, Haiti, India, and Thailand.

While there may be no vaccine against it yet, malaria can be prevented. Prophylactic drugs—medicines taken before exposure to the disease to protect against it—are an effective guard against malaria. Most often, travelers to areas where malaria is endemic will be given the drug chloroquine (Aralen), which helps ward off the most lethal type of malaria, called *P. falciparum*. To be effective, chloroquine should be taken starting a week or two before traveling to an area with malaria, and should be continued for six weeks after leaving.

In some parts of the world, there have been strains of malaria reported that are resistant to chloroquine. Travelers to these areas may be given the drug combination sulfadoxine and pyrimethamine, sold under the brand name Fansidar, in addition to chloroquine. It, too, is taken starting a week or two before traveling to a malaria-infested area, and is continued for six weeks after departure. Fansidar's use is still controversial, however, because of severe side effects and complications, including deaths, that have been reported. Anyone taking the drug who notices a skin rash should stop taking the medication immediately and report the symptom to a physician. And anyone taking the drug over a prolonged period should have regular blood counts and urine analysis to make sure the drug is not having any harmful effects.

Fansidar is now usually given presumptively, meaning that it is taken along on a trip and then only used after symptoms of illness, including fever, appear. Fansidar is only recommended preventively for travelers who will be spending three weeks or longer in an area with a high rate of chloroquine-resistant malaria transmission. A third drug—primaquine—may be prescribed to treat or prevent the symptoms of another type of malaria, called *P. vivax* or relapsing malaria, after you leave an endemic area and return home.

Know that you can still get malaria even if you take preventive medication. And any symptoms of headache, malaise, fever, chills, or sweats following travel to a malaria-endemic area (even up to months afterward) should be investigated by a physician.

Travelers can also minimize their chances of getting malaria—as well as any of the other approximately eighty mosquito-borne diseases and countless illnesses transmitted by fleas, ticks, flies, and other insects—by sleeping in air-conditioned hotel rooms with closed windows, or under mosquito netting. Using insect repellents (those containing N,N-diethyl-meta-toluamide, also known as DEET, are considered the most effective), wearing light-colored clothing that covers the arms and legs, staying inside or covering up after dark, and avoiding strong cologne or aftershave will also help keep insects away.

The good news for travelers is that researchers are working on perfecting a malaria vaccine. The Food and Drug Administration is studying the data, and within the next five to ten years chloroquine and Fansidar treatment may be things of the past.

Information Sources

A country-by-country guide to immunization and malaria conditions is included in chapter 14, but the risk of acquiring a specific disease in a specific area changes rapidly—there may be a malaria epidemic one month, and a yellow fever epidemic the next, for example—so it's important to check out your destination shortly before you leave.

Don't rely on your travel agent or tour leader for medical advice. Most are unaware of all the health hazards for any given country. The first place you should call for information is your federal, state, or local health department. Your physician can also call for you. These government health departments regularly receive the latest information from the Centers for Disease Control in Atlanta, and the World Health Organization in Geneva; they can pass that information directly on to you. An alternative would be for your physician to contact the Travelers' Health Activity at the Centers for Disease Control in Atlanta, to inquire directly about the proper precautions for a specific destination; the number is (404) 329-2572. In addition to these sources, there are other services—some free, some that charge a fee:

■ **Immunization Alert™.** Immunization Alert™ is a new, computerized information service. Physicians, state and local health departments, corporations, and medical schools can subscribe, and receive periodic computer diskettes with up-to-date information on the health conditions and immunization requirements and recommendations for over two hundred countries. If your company or physician does not subscribe, you can still request information on a specific destination. For a fee—currently $30—you can obtain a computer printout of the health conditions and recommended immunizations for up to six countries. Each additional country costs $10. Immunization Alert™ gets its information from the Centers for Disease Control, the World Health Organization, and the U.S. State Department. The computer's data base is updated daily to reflect changing conditions. For more information, write to Kenneth R. Dardick, M.D., Medical Director, Immunization Alert, P.O. Box 406, Storrs, CT 06268. Telephone: (203) 487-0422.

■ **State Department Overseas Citizens' Emergency Center.** This government service, located in Washington, D.C., will provide information by phone on current epidemics and health conditions around the world. The line is answered from Monday through Friday, 8:15 A.M. to 10:00 P.M. Eastern time. The number is (202) 647-5225.

If you do become ill when traveling, this number can also be used by friends and relatives to obtain information on your condition, and to help you arrange medical evacuation home if necessary. Nights, weekends, and in real emergencies, call (202) 647-1512 or (202) 634-3600. Make sure that someone back home always has a complete copy of your itinerary, including flight numbers, hotel addresses, and phone numbers, and exact dates of when you'll be where. And write or send a telegram home if there are any changes as you travel.

■ **Worldwide Health Forecast.** Run by HealthCare Abroad, a travel insurance company (see next section), this is another phone service that maintains information on world health conditions. The toll-free number is: (800) 368-3531.

■ **International Association for Medical Assistance to Travelers (IAMAT).** A nonprofit foundation, IAMAT maintains lists of American and English-speaking physicians abroad, as well as up-to-date health information (including weather, safety of food and water, local diseases, and immunization requirements) for locations around the world. IAMAT membership is free, although a donation is suggested, and entitles the user to the list of English-speaking doctors. These doctors have agreed to charge IAMAT members only $20 for an office visit, $30 for a visit to a hotel or home, and $35 for a call at night, on Sundays, or on local holidays. Members also receive a series of pamphlets, including immunization guides and advice on preventing disease. With a donation of $25 or more, IAMAT will send travelers a set of 24 charts of climate, food, and water conditions for about 1,400 cities worldwide. IAMAT will even provide travelers with packets of oral rehydration salts (Dialite) to help cope with diarrhea. For more information, write: IAMAT, 417 Center Street, Lewiston, NY 14092, or call (716) 754-4883, from Monday through Friday, 9 A.M. to 5 P.M. Eastern time.

■ **Intermedic.** Membership in Intermedic—which costs $6 per individual and $10 per family for one year—entitles the cardholder to a list of English-speaking doctors abroad. These physicians have agreed to charge members no more than $40 for an initial office visit, $50 for an initial house or hotel visit, and $60 for a house or hotel visit at night. Intermedic also provides an Overseas Health Information Service, which answers queries about immunizations and medications. For more information, write: Intermedic, Inc., 777 Third Avenue, New York, NY 10017, or call (212) 486-8900.

■ **Banana Republic's Climate Desk.** This national chain of clothing stores now staffs a phone line with operators who can provide information on over five hundred destinations. They can tell you about a given locale's temperature and humidity, give you an update on the current political situation, and even recommend what clothing to pack. The Climate Desk can also provide health and immunization information. Call (800) 325-7270, Monday through Friday, 8:30 A.M. to 5:00 P.M. Pacific time.

Travelers' Medical Insurance: Protection for Your Body and Your Wallet

One final thing to think about before you leave. If you've followed the advice in this chapter so far, you've done a lot to protect yourself against illness while traveling. But in spite of the best precautions, there's no guarantee that you won't get sick or be involved in an accident. So the next health decision you have to make before you leave is whether to protect your finances in case of illness away from home.

The first assumption that many travelers make, which is only partially correct, is that their company health plan or personal insurance will cover them in the event of illness abroad. Read your policy carefully—it may very well be true. But what is not mentioned anywhere is the fact that if you're treated by a foreign doctor or hospital, they may not want to wait for reimbursement from an American insurance company. They may demand that you pay them immediately, and that *you* wait to be reimbursed by the company. Some foreign hospitals may even withhold a patient's passport until the bill is paid . . . in cash or travelers' checks (although some big city hospitals overseas now accept credit cards). How many travelers carry enough money to cover a medical emergency? And for senior citizens, Medicare does not cover medical expenses incurred abroad, except in Canada and Mexico. (Senior citizens with Medicare who want to obtain supplemental coverage for travel outside the U.S. can contact the American Association of Retired Persons [AARP] Insurance; (800) 523-5800. In Pennsylvania call (800) 492-2024.)

Companies specializing in policies for travelers make arrangements for immediate and direct payment, so you don't have to worry about not being able to pay a medical bill. Anyone who suffers from a medical condition that may need attention abroad, who is elderly, who will be away for an extended period of time, or who is traveling with children, should seriously consider investing in a travelers' health policy. Think of it as temporary major medical coverage.

Before you invest in a travelers' insurance policy, check to see what kind of services your credit card company offers. American Express Platinum Card holders and Gold MasterCard holders receive travel emergency-assistance coverage, including medical insurance, as part of their membership benefits. And while regular American Express cardholders do not receive travelers' medical insurance as a membership benefit, they can take advantage of a service called Global Assist. An emergency referral service, Global Assist helps provide world travelers with advice by phone, twenty-four hours a day. The advice includes information about inoculations; help in finding a doctor, dentist, or pharmacist; shipment of prescription medications abroad; even sending messages to friends and relatives. People who purchase BankAmerica Travelers Cheques have the option of joining the Safe-Travel Network. The $5 cost entitles the buyer to medical insurance, access to a 24-hour emergency phone number, plus a worldwide network of physicians, and other services. Coverage lasts for 45 days. More and more banks and credit card companies will probably be adding travelers' services to their list of benefits; call your credit card company when you're planning a trip to find out if you have any travel health coverage through them.

If you decide you need additional coverage, investigate policies and check the restrictions carefully—make sure you know when, and under what circumstances, an illness or injury will be covered. For instance, some companies will not provide coverage in countries, such as El Salvador, considered politically dangerous for Americans. Many companies specifically exclude chronic illnesses from their coverage, an important point for people with health conditions. Most policies also exclude third trimester pregnancy; many exclude sports-related injuries (for example, scuba or ski accidents).

Also check to see if you are covered in the United States as well as abroad, if the company provides help or merely reimbursement (this is very important, since the company's expert help—medical advice and translation services—in an emergency can be every bit as valuable as the fees they pay for you), if there is a limit on the amount they will pay, what kind of medical documentation is necessary for reimbursement, and how quickly they can provide help in an emergency.

What most of the companies *do* provide: twenty-four-hour hotlines staffed by operators who will find American doctors to give advice, locate the nearest English-speaking physician abroad and contact relatives or family doctors; emergency evacuation back to the United States; *some* payment coverage for medical costs; and help in replacing prescription medicines abroad. Some companies will even fly a family member to visit the insured party in the hospital, or provide a traveling companion for children should their parent(s) or guardian(s) become ill. Many companies will even cover the cost of your trip if you are forced to cancel for medical reasons.

Most companies offer their protection on a per-trip or weekly basis: The cost varies, but is generally $20 to $50 a week. For frequent travelers, many companies offer an annual membership for around $200.

Check your personal insurance company; they may offer a special plan for travelers themselves. If not, the following are the names and addresses of some companies which offer special travelers' insurance policies:

- Access America Inc., a subsidiary of Blue Cross and Blue Shield of the Washington, D.C. and New York area, 600 Third Avenue, Box 807, New York, NY 10163. Telephone: (800) 851-2800 between 8 A.M. and 6 P.M., Monday through Friday, Eastern time; all other times call (800) 654-6686.
- Air-Evac International, 8665 Gibbs Drive, Suite 202, San Diego, CA 92123. Telephone: (800) 854-2569. In California call (619) 292-5557.
- ARM Coverage Inc., Box 310, 120 Mineola Boulevard, Mineola, NY 11501. Telephone: (800) 645-2424. In New York call (516) 294-0220.
- Global Assistance Network, 999 Summer Street, Stamford, CT 06905. Telephone: (800) 368-2110. In Connecticut call (203) 964-9137.

- Healthcare Abroad, Suite 219 Investment Building, 1511 K St. N.W., Washington, D.C. 20005. Telephone: (800) 336-3310. In Virginia call (703) 255-9800.
- International Medical Systems, 3 Waters Park Drive, Suite 217, San Mateo, CA 94403. Telephone: (800) 862-9900. In California call (415) 571-0611.
- International SOS Assistance Inc., P.O. Box 11568, Philadelphia, PA 19116. Telephone: (800) 523-8930. In Pennsylvania call (215) 244-1500.
- Mutual of Omaha Travel Insurance, Tele-Trip Co. Inc., 3201 Farnam St., Omaha, NE 68131. Telephone: (800) 228-9792. In Nebraska call (402) 342-7600 or 345-2400.
- Travel Assistance International: 1333 F Street N.W., Suite 300, Washington, D.C. 20004. Telephone: (800) 821-2828. In the District of Columbia call (202) 347-2025.
- Travel Guard International, 1100 Centerpoint Drive, Stevens Point, WI 54481. Telephone: (800) 826-1300. In Wisconsin call (715) 346-6000 or 345-0505.
- The Travelers Insurance Companies, c/o Travel Pak, One Tower Square, Hartford, CT 06183-5040. Telephone: (800) 243-3174. In Connecticut call (203) 277-0111.
- Travel Protection Plan, Confidence/Riebling & Co., 25 Ann St., New York, NY 10038. Telephone: (800) 221-5564. In New York call (212) 962-2602. Or inquire at any American Express Vacation Store.
- TravMed-Medex, Box 10623, Baltimore, MD 21204. Telephone: (800) 732-5309. In Maryland call (301) 296-5225.
- World Access Inc., Suite 200, 2115 Ward Court N.W., Washington, D.C. 20037. Telephone: (800) 482-0016. In Washington, D.C. call (202) 822-3978.
- WorldCare Travel Assistance Association, 2000 Pennsylvania Avenue N.W., Suite 7600, Washington, D.C. 20006. Telephone: (800) 521-4822. In the District of Columbia call (202) 293-0335.

2 | Transportation R$_x$

You've made your plans, you've packed your clothes, and you can't wait to hit the beach, visit every museum in London, photograph every lion in Kenya, or wow the chairman of the board of Japan's largest electronics firm. But in spite of your preparations, you still have to get there. And for many travelers, the flight, cruise, train, bus, or car ride can be the most grueling ordeal of all.

Jet lag, motion sickness, sea sickness, popping ear drums, and just plain stiff limbs and swollen ankles from sitting too long, all can spoil the mood of even the most anticipated journey. Once again, there's no reason to put up with these discomforts. For each travel woe, there is a soothing solution.

Jilting Jet Lag

Traveling to far-off places unfortunately means crossing time zones . . . and that usually means jet lag. When your body's clock is suddenly reset, you feel jet lag's symptoms: fatigue, insomnia, indigestion, headaches, irritability, and general disorientation. These collective symptoms are called "jet lag" because airplane travel is primarily responsible for the phenomenon; before the age of air travel, it took long enough to travel from one place to another that the body had time to adjust to new time zones during the journey. But airplanes make it possible to cross many time zones in a day or less, wreaking havoc on the body's clock.

Individuals differ in their susceptibility to symptoms of jet lag. Scientists are not sure why, but in general, younger travelers feel less discomfort and adjust more quickly to changes in time zones. Most people find it easier to adjust when traveling westward—for instance, from Paris to New York—when the time difference means an extension of the first day. Eastward travel—New York to Paris—cuts the first day short and drastically compresses the day/night cycle, disrupting sleep patterns.

A general rule to follow in dealing with jet lag is: Allow one day to adjust for every time zone you cross (in other words, for every hour of time difference). That's not a problem if you're traveling from New York to Chicago with a one-hour difference; in fact, many people will not really feel the effects of jet lag unless they cross at least three time zones. Flying to Asia, where the time difference is a half day or more, however, will be baffling to your body, accustomed as it is to regular meal times and sleeping hours. Even a trip to Europe, with about a six-hour time difference from New York, takes travelers about a week from which to recover.

And it's not just eating and sleeping patterns that are disrupted by crossing time zones. Alertness, temperature, athletic prowess, sexual moods, decisiveness, and many other mental and physical abilities are affected by jet lag.

Luckily, you don't have to spend the better part of your business trip or vacation wide-awake in the middle of the night or dead tired at noon, because there are several ways to prevent jet lag, or at least to ease its symptoms. The traveler willing to put some effort into jilting jet lag a few days before his or her trip will find the symptoms greatly reduced.

Body rhythms are programmed by factors called zeitgebers (German for "time-givers"), internal and external stimuli that help set the body's clock. Zeitgebers include light, work schedules, food, alcohol, caffeine, exercise, mental stimulation, and social activity. Jet lag can be combated by altering any of these zeitgebers, but the three basic strategies for easing jet lag are changing sleep, diet, or light.

Read the descriptions of each method below and decide which one will best fit into your pre-trip schedule.

SLEEP

The most obvious way to prevent jet lag—but probably the least convenient—is to alter your sleeping hours gradually, while you're still home, to conform to those of your destination. If you're traveling to Europe, try to go to sleep an hour earlier each night for about a week. By the time you leave, you might be going to sleep at 6:00 P.M. your time, but it will be about midnight in Europe. Change your meal times, too, to correspond with your new hours. By forcing yourself to live on

European time before you even get there, you'll fit right in when you do.

Unfortunately, this method is nearly impossible for anyone with a job, a family, or a social life. Still, even if you can't change your schedule completely before you leave, altering it by even one or two hours will make the adjustment easier when you arrive.

Skip the evening news and go to sleep an hour earlier, for example; then wake up an hour earlier and catch the morning news instead. It may seem like a small change, but it will save you one full day of adjusting if you're traveling east. Conversely, if you're traveling west, try to stay up and watch a late movie or talk show. Shower, wash your hair, lay out your clothes for the next day, and fill the coffeepot in advance so you can sleep an hour later in the morning. Again, you'll save yourself a full day of adjusting by this small change if you're traveling west.

DIET

By following a special anti-jet lag diet developed by Dr. Charles F. Ehret of the Argonne National Laboratory in Argonne, Illinois, a traveler can ease the symptoms of jet lag considerably. The diet should be followed for three days before flying.

The medical theory behind the diet is a bit complicated—it is based on the belief that jet lag is due not only to fatigue, but to desynchronization of the body's organs. The diet helps "reset" the organs by depleting and replenishing the liver's supply of glycogen. Some experts, however, feel the diet works because the people following it have put enough time and energy into the diet that they *believe* it will work. Whatever the reason, the important thing is that the diet *does* work. By alternating "feast" and "fast" days (the pattern in which they're alternated depends on which direction you're flying) you can help set your body's natural rhythms for your destination before you arrive.

The diet's biggest advantage is its proven effectiveness, but drawbacks include its relative complexity, and the fact that it requires you to change your eating habits and plan your meals carefully right before your departure—a time when you will obviously be busy packing and taking care of last-minute details for your trip. The effort is certainly worthwhile for business travelers, and for vacationers who don't want to miss a minute of sightseeing because of fatigue. But for pleasure seekers headed to warm climes and a tranquil beach, it might just be worth it to let the sun, the sand, and the palm trees take care of the jet lag for you.

To follow the anti-jet lag diet:

Start the diet three days before your departure day. These three days are the same whether you are traveling east or west. The first day of the diet is a "feast" day, which means you should eat a high protein (meats, eggs, cereals and beans) breakfast and lunch, and a high carbohydrate (pasta, potatoes, starchy vegetables, sweet desserts) supper. Keep protein servings very small at supper.

The second day of the diet is a "fast" day. You don't have to avoid eating completely, but keep meals small and low in calories and carbohydrates. Try to limit your food intake to fruit, light soups, broths, skimpy salads, dry toast.

On the third day, you can once again "feast" as on the first day. Throughout these three days limit your intake of caffeinated beverages, such as coffee, tea, and some soft drinks, to between the hours of 3 P.M. and 5 P.M.

Finally, on the day of departure, fast again. If you're traveling west, you may drink caffeinated beverages early in the morning; your fast will only be for half a day. If you're traveling east, you may drink caffeinated beverages between 6 P.M. and 11 P.M.; your fast will be for the entire day.

On the airplane, avoid alcohol completely. If your flight is long enough, try to sleep until your destination's breakfast time, *but no later*. No matter which direction you're traveling, break your fast at your destination's breakfast time by eating a high protein breakfast. (This is a crucial part of the diet. You may want to ask the flight attendant to hold your supper until breakfast time. Another option: bring high protein foods such as cheese or peanut butter along with you to be sure of breaking the fast correctly.)

The day of your arrival (which may be the same day as your departure day if you're traveling west) is a "feast" day, so you will eat a high protein lunch and a high carbohydrate supper after you arrive. Eat these meals at the times that are normal for your destination, and don't let yourself fall asleep until it is evening there. When you wake up the next morning, your body should be accustomed to the new time.

If you don't have the time or the inclination to follow the diet completely, follow an abbreviated version by starting on the day of your departure with a "fast" day. Continue following the diet on the airplane and after arrival. It may not be as effective as the complete diet, but it will still help shorten your adjustment time.

Details of Dr. Ehret's diet are contained in the book *Overcoming Jet Lag* by Dr. Charles F. Ehret and Lynne Waller Scanlon (Berkley Books, 1983). For a wallet-sized card describing the diet, send a self-addressed, stamped envelope to: Anti-Jet Lag Diet, OPA, Argonne National Laboratory, 9700 South Cass Avenue, Argonne, IL 60439.

LIGHT

Light is considered the primary zeitgeber, and one of the newest theories on dealing with jet lag involves altering the amount and hours of light exposure. Dr. Alfred Lewy of the Oregon Health Sciences University in Portland has studied the effects of daylight on the hormone melatonin, which may be the body's main timekeeper. (In fact, preliminary studies in England have shown that melatonin, taken in pill form, can prevent jet lag. Soon an anti-jet lag pill of melatonin may be available to the public.)

Dr. Lewy recommends that travelers take advantage of natural light when they reach their destination to help their bodies adjust to a new time zone. West to east travelers crossing six or less time zones should get a few hours of early morning light (it must be outdoor, not indoor, light) for the first few days after arrival. The more time zones you've crossed (up to six), the more hours of daylight you should try to catch. An easy rule of thumb: Try to expose yourself to at least as many hours of light as the number of time zones you've crossed. But if you've crossed six to twelve time zones, stay indoors early and get your sunlight later in the day.

East to west travelers (also crossing six or less time zones) should go outside in the late afternoon the day of arrival and for a few days afterward, for a few hours. Again, the more time zones crossed (up to six), the more hours you should spend in the light. If you cross six to twelve time zones westward, avoid sunlight toward the end of the day.

The idea is that by exposing the body to light during unaccustomed hours, you can reset your body's clock so that you'll be able to adjust more quickly to the sleeping and waking hours of a new environment. (A few words of advice: Consider wearing a sunscreen to protect your skin, and avoid looking directly at the sun so as not to injure your eyes.) This method even works on a rainy or overcast day—but the light *must* come from outdoors, not indoors.

While Dr. Lewy cautions that this method is still experimental, its advantages are that it requires no special foods, drugs, or other alteration of your eating and sleeping habits. Depending on how flexible your travel schedule is, of course, you may find it difficult to fit the hours of light exposure into your itinerary.

If you're a natural procrastinator or if all the above simply sounds like too much of an effort, there are a few things you can do on the day of your flight, during your flight, or even after your arrival to ease jet lag discomfort.

First of all, make sure you start out on your trip as relaxed and well-rested as possible (difficult, to be sure, since most vacationers are going away expressly to relax, and most business travelers won't be able to relax either before or during their trips). Try to avoid planning demanding activities for the day you arrive.

As soon as you board the plane, set your watch for the time zone of your destination. Try as much as possible to adopt immediately the local meal schedules—in other words, if the flight attendant serves you a large meal—dinner—when you know it's breakfasttime where you're headed, try to eat as close to what you would normally eat at breakfast as possible. For instance, have the roll and coffee, and leave the chicken and vegetables.

If you're traveling to Europe, consider taking a day flight instead of the all-too-common overnight flights. When your flight lands, it will be evening in Europe. Go to sleep soon after arrival and try to sleep through the night. The next day, immediately adopt the local eating and sleeping hours. If a daytime flight isn't possible, and your flight arrives in Europe early in the morning, try to force yourself to stay awake through the day, and eat lunch and dinner at the local times. If you absolutely must nap during the day, try to keep the nap short—no longer than one or two hours. Don't rely on alcohol or tranquilizers to help you sleep, or caffeine to keep you awake. These will only confuse your body further.

Keep snacks on hand in your hotel room, since you may wake up in the middle of the first few nights ravenously hungry (you will also probably wake up and have to use the bathroom). And be prepared to suffer more the second night than the first, since the fatigue most people feel from traveling helps them sleep the first night.

If you're really too lazy to make any special effort to ease jet lag, ask your doctor about prescribing a short-acting sleeping pill, such as triazolam (Halcion) to help you sleep on an overnight flight, or for the first few nights after you arrive. Joint studies at Stanford University Medical Center and the Henry Ford Hospital in Detroit found that short-acting drugs can be helpful. Your physician can recommend the proper drug for you.

The Joy of Movement

Rolling ships, rocking airplanes, and lurching automobiles can turn even the most seasoned traveler green. If you suffer from motion sickness, you're not alone. Experts estimate that one out of twenty people consistently experiences motion sickness, while at least nine out of ten of the rest of us will react to especially bumpy, jerky, or rough rides.

How can you tell whether you'll be one of the unlucky sufferers? First of all, there is an age factor. Children under two and adults over fifty are the least likely to suffer from motion sickness, while children between two and twelve are the most likely to experience it. Joggers and swimmers seem to be less susceptible to motion sickness, since their bodies are accustomed to movement. Interestingly, deaf people are virtually immune to motion sickness, because their inner ears—the body's balance center—do not function properly.

If traveling from point A to point B consistently turns you green, you should know that about half of NASA astronauts and even animals such as fish and dogs share your problem. In fact, NASA scientists are conducting much of the research into new cures for motion sickness. Even now, however, there are plenty of ways to help your body adapt.

You probably think you know the symptoms of motion sickness: nausea and vomiting. But these are actually the *final* symptoms. Before them may come facial paleness, yawning, restlessness, and a cold sweat. These symptoms may progress to drowsiness and an upset stomach—by this time, the unlucky traveler usually knows what's in store. What causes these symptoms, culminating in the final race for the deck rail or the airsickness bag?

Motion sickness, scientists believe, occurs when the eyes and ears get conflicting messages about movement. For instance, your inner ear, which registers movement and controls balance, may feel the movement of an automobile, but your eyes are focused on the pages of a stationary book or magazine. What scientists aren't yet sure of, is why a sensory problem such as this causes gastrointestinal problems—in other words, why a communications problem between your eyes and your ears affects your stomach.

In time, many people actually outgrow motion sickness; their bodies learn to deal with the conflicting signals. But others do not. And, as mentioned before, a rough enough ride will affect virtually everyone, as may a new experience, such as the first time on a boat or plane.

Right now, the easiest way to deal with motion sickness is to prevent it. Start by choosing your traveling position carefully.

■ In an automobile, the best position is the driver's seat. Car drivers almost never get carsick, because since they're controlling the automobile, they anticipate its movements. If you can't be the driver, the next best thing is to sit in the front seat next to him so you're aware of what he's doing. Don't snack in the car, and keep a window open for fresh air. (*Always* wear a seat belt; the pressure around your middle is not enough to aggravate nausea.)

■ On a bus, try to sit toward the front, near a (preferably open) window. If possible, you should be able to see the driver, and out the front window, too, so you can anticipate the bus's movements a bit.

■ On a train you have an important choice to make: Sit facing forward, near a window, to help prevent motion sickness. (Focus on a distant point on the horizon, rather than on something in the vehicle or whizzing by right outside it.) But some trains have seats facing backward, and studies show that these seats are safest in the—admittedly unlikely—event of a crash.

■ On an airplane, the seats over the wings or wheels are the most stable. The tail section is the bumpiest. (Again, a choice to be made: The areas near the wings are also the most susceptible to fire because the fuselage is under the wings.) Keep the air vents over your seat open, directed toward your face. And relax; of all forms of transportation, you are least likely to get motion sick on a plane.

■ On a boat, try to get a midships cabin, one or two decks below the public rooms (close to the waterline). Spend as much time as possible out on deck in the fresh air. Avoid reading if you know you tend to suffer from motion sickness.

You can also improve your chances by not eating a heavy meal right before your trip . . . you don't want to give your stomach another problem with which to cope. During a long trip, forego large meals and greasy foods in favor of frequent, light snacks. Avoid alcohol and strong odors such as tobacco smoke. Be well rested before your trip. Wear loose clothing for comfort. One of the best things you can do is relax—anxiety about motion sickness unfortunately improves your chances of developing it. And the power of suggestion is a strong one: If you notice other people on your plane or boat getting sick, try not to stay around them.

If experience has taught you that in spite of anything you do, you will get carsick, airsick, or seasick (not everyone who suffers from one will suffer from another—seasickness is by far the most common), consider motion sickness medication. Even if you don't normally suffer from motion sickness, you may want to take medication to prevent it if the seas are especially rough, or if the plane may be encountering a great deal of air turbulence.

The most common medications are the over-the-counter antihistamines: cyclizine hydrochloride (Marezine), meclizine hydrochloride (Bonine), and dimenhydrinate (Dramamine). The drugs work best when taken from thirty to sixty minutes before traveling. Once nausea begins, it's usually too late for the drugs to work (for one thing, many people will vomit—and expel the drugs—before they can take effect). Asthmatics, persons with glaucoma, and those with enlargement of the prostate should *not* take these medications. Check the package instructions or ask your physician for more information. The drawback of all these medicines is that because they are antihistamines, they may cause drowsiness.

There are also antinausea and antivomiting prescription drugs that are effective against motion sickness. The most popular is scopolamine. As an oral medication, the drug can cause side effects such as drowsiness, dryness of the mouth, blurred vision, a sensitivity to light, and heart irregularities. (NASA gives astronauts scopolamine in combination with a stimulant to combat motion sickness.) But scopolamine is now available as a dime-sized patch, worn behind the ear, to minimize the side effects. The drug is absorbed through the thin skin behind the ear, and enters the bloodstream at a slow, steady rate. It's applied two to four hours before traveling, and lasts for three days. A definite improvement over oral scopolamine, the patch (brand name Transderm Scōp) may still produce some of the side effects listed above. Anyone who uses the patch should wash his hands after applying it, since there is medication on the adhesive, which, when transferred from hand to eye, can cause pupil dilation. Also, the patch should not be used by children, people with glaucoma, or those with urinary or bowel obstruction. The patch should only be used with caution by the elderly.

Old wives' tales and home remedies for motion sickness include sucking a lemon, pressing an acupuncture point on the inside of the wrist, and swallowing capsules of ground ginger (available in many health food stores). Some recent studies have shown that ginger is effective. If you'd like to try ginger instead of medication (one advantage is that it won't make you sleepy), try swallowing two ginger capsules about fifteen minutes before traveling. Take more whenever necessary, since it's nearly impossible to overdose: You'll know when you've taken more than you need by a slight burning sensation in the upper chest/throat.

Once the symptoms of motion sickness begin, they are difficult to stop. Since swallowing drugs is of little use when a person is vomiting, physicians will give injections or suppositories of motion sickness medication in severe cases. But before resorting to drastic measures, try mind-over-body programming, since there is a strong psychological component to motion sickness.

1). Breathe slowly and deeply with your mouth open (fresh air, if possible) until the nausea subsides.

2). Stare at a fixed spot directly in front of you (in the direction the vehicle is moving), blocking out all other stimuli.

3). Concentrate on tensing your body, and then slowly relaxing all the muscles. Repeat the action rhythmically until you feel better.

4). Either seek a quiet spot where you can lie down and rest, or get absorbed in some kind of recreation or activity and focus on that.

Other strategies for calming a motion-sick stomach include: lying down with the eyes closed, holding the head as still as possible, and eating dry crackers. Whether or not the above methods help your queasy stomach, take comfort in the fact that most people do adapt to new motion within a couple of days, and symptoms will eventually subside on their own. If motion sickness lasts for several days, see a physician. You might not be suffering from motion sickness at all, but from food poisoning or some other stomach disorder.

For now, the ideal motion sickness drug does not exist. The perfect drug could be taken after symptoms appear, and it would have no side effects at all. Such a drug does not even appear to be on the horizon. But there is research being done into new medications for motion sickness, and a new European drug, manufactured by Janssen Pharmaceutica in Belgium and called Touristil (a combination of cinnarizine, which is a European drug used to treat vertigo, and domperidone, an antiemetic) may eventually be available in the United States. Like most of the drugs now available, it, too, must be taken preventively. But unlike other anti-motion sickness medications, it does not cause drowsiness. And NASA is developing a biofeedback technique called Autogenic Feedback Training that may eventually prove more effective than any currently available drug.

Traveling in Comfort

Why do people always seem to lurch bleary-eyed off planes, stumble off boats and drag themselves out of cars, buses, and trains? Probably because they didn't know how to keep themselves comfortable. What you eat, what you drink, and your level of activity all affect how you'll feel by the end of the voyage. So does the clothing you wear. Whether you're traveling by plane, train, bus, or ship, you should wear loose, comfortable clothing that is not restrictive. Your movement will be limited enough in most vehicle seats; don't make yourself even more uncomfortable by wearing tight pants or a snug, button-down collar. It's also a good idea to dress in layers, so you can adjust your clothing to match the temperature on board.

Beyond this general advice, here are some specific tips for helping you arrive at your destination cool, calm, collected, and relaxed, no matter what the conveyance.

AIRPLANE

You'll probably have to try to keep yourself comfortable on an airplane in spite of the airlines and the flight attendants, not because of them. Terrible food, uncomfortable seats, and stale, dry air are hardly conducive to a pleasant flight.

The first thing to do is ignore the flight attendants plying you with alcohol, coffee, and carbonated soft drinks. All these beverages are actually dehydrating, and their effect is increased by the dryness of the cabin air. Also, caffeinated drinks will aggravate jet lag by affecting your sleep on the flight. Carbonated soft drinks can make you uncomfortable when the air pressure in the cabin changes . . . and the gas from the soda expands in your digestive tract.

Instead, ask for water or fruit juice, and lots of it, to compensate for the dryness. Since many airlines only carry enough juice to use as mixers, you may want to bring your own juice or bottles of mineral water on board with you. If possible, also try to avoid eating large meals or smoking during a flight, since they add to fatigue and stress on the body. (You can request special meals—including Kosher, low salt, low calorie, diabetic, vegetarian, low cholesterol, and so forth—on many airlines. Just be sure to give them at least twenty-four hours' notice.)

In addition to the loose, layered clothing you're wearing, make sure your shoes are also loose and comfortable. Sneakers or soft shoes that expand comfortably with your feet are best. Keep them on throughout the flight. *Don't* wear tight shoes and take them off when you sit down—you may find them impossible to put back on when the flight lands. Most people's feet and ankles swell during a long flight. The condition is caused by the altered pressure and gravitational pull, as well as the inactivity of plane travel, forcing blood to the extremities. Wearing support stockings may help. Don't sit with your legs crossed, since it will reduce the circulation to your legs even further. Sometimes, passengers suffer discomfort in their legs because of the cabin floor's vibrations. Placing a blanket beneath your feet or periodically raising your feet off the floor may help.

Sitting still during a long flight makes many people restless and uncomfortable; it can also aggravate the symptoms of jet lag. In response to the national fitness craze, and an increasingly mobile population, many airlines now offer in-flight exercise tapes and pamphlets for those who want a structured workout to help fill the time and make them feel better. Some of the programs now available:

- Japan Air Lines offers a ten-minute stretch program that is screened at regular intervals during their flights.
- Lufthansa German Airlines has published a "Fitness in the Chair" brochure. The pamphlet is not distributed in-flight, but you can send for it by enclosing a self-addressed envelope and writing to: Lufthansa, Dept. UX112, 1640 Hempstead Turnpike, East Meadow, NY 11544.
- SAS (Scandinavian Airlines System) publishes a booklet called "Exercise in the Chair" with descriptions of in-seat stretches and exercises. Again, the pamphlet is not provided on board, but you can send for it by writing to: SAS, Execu-Stretch, 825 Third Avenue, Suite 3300, New York, NY 10022.

If your flight doesn't offer an "airplane aerobics" program, you can bring one on board yourself. The staff at the Capitol Hill Hospital Sports Medicine Program in Washington, D.C., together with the Washington Healthcare Corporation, has developed a thirty-minute in-flight exercise program. Available on a standard cassette, the program can be used by anyone who brings his own cassette player on board. The cassette, which features fifteen minutes of isometric exercises and fifteen minutes of relaxation exercises, costs $6.95, and is available from Fitness in Flight, Washington Healthcare Corp., East Building, Suite 8102, 100 Irving Street N.W., Washington, D.C. 20010.

If your flight doesn't offer an "airplane aerobics" program, and you haven't brought one on board, there are some simple exercises you can do on your own which work almost as well. You should try both to walk around the cabin and do these exercises at least once every other hour, and again an hour before landing.

1). Try tensing and relaxing your muscles, one by one. Suck your stomach in, hold for a count of five, then release it. Clench your fists, then let go. Contract your buttocks, then relax. Repeat.

2). Concentrate on moving every joint in your body. Start by wiggling your toes, then rotating your ankles, bending your knees, etc.

3). If you're lucky enough to have an empty seat next to you, pretend you're rowing a boat. Grasp the imaginary oars, lean forward, then slowly rotate your arms and shoulders.

4). Shrug your shoulders by raising them as high as you can, holding the position for a count of five, then lowering them. Roll your shoulders forward and backward, then your head from side to side (gently, to prevent neck injury).

5). Reach one arm overhead and stretch toward the ceiling, as if there were something up there you wanted to grab. Repeat with other arm.

6). Breathe deeply as much as possible throughout the flight. Inhale through your nose, and exhale through your mouth (with lips pursed in a silent whistle).

Your skin also suffers during a long plane ride; the dry cabin air in jet planes (with a relative humidity of only about 10 percent) can make it feel rough and scaly, your hair limp and flyaway. Put some sample size bottles of facial moisturizer, hand cream, and lip balm in your carry-on bag, and use them periodically during the flight. (Several companies now make cosmetic creams specially formulated to combat the dry skin caused by cabin air. Prescriptives' Flight Cream and Orlane's Hydro-Climat are two of these. Besides hydrating the skin, they also help avoid the pasty, pale, tired look that most of us have after a long trip.) Carry a mineral water spray—you can fill an atomizer yourself— to spritz on your face underneath your moisturizer. Also, condition your hair before a long flight to prevent it from drying out.

If you wear either hard or soft contact lenses, carry plenty of lubricating drops on board and use them frequently to prevent dry eyes; make sure you remove your lenses for even the shortest nap. This is a good idea even for people with extended-wear lenses. And if you have problems with nosebleeds exacerbated by dry air, use a lubricating jelly such as Vaseline inside your nostrils before the flight.

One last problem often stops people from enjoying a flight—that horrible sensation of your ears aching, crackling, and popping in reaction to the altered pressure. The problem is usually worst during descent, when the air pressure in the plane is greater than the pressure inside your ears. To keep your ears pain-free, you must try to equalize the pressure. Some ways of dealing with this problem: sipping liquids, sucking on hard candies, chewing gum, yawning, or opening your mouth wide. Try not to sleep during takeoff and landing, since you won't swallow frequently enough to keep your ears clear. Another good method, called the modified Valsalva's maneuver, is to pinch your nostrils shut with your fingers, take a mouthful of air, then use your cheek and throat muscles to force the air into the back of the nose, as if you were trying to blow your thumb and fingers off your nostrils. (It's important not to use your lungs or diaphragm to force the air, but only your cheek and throat muscles. Too high pressures could cause dizziness and fainting, and interfere with circulation.) A loud pop in the ears signals success. You may have to repeat the modified Valsalva's maneuver several times during the flight to keep your ears unclogged.

If you always suffer from this problem, or if you're flying with a cold (which should be avoided whenever possible, since it is very uncomfortable, and can make the cold much worse), consider taking a decongestant tablet or using a decongestant nasal spray an hour before takeoff, and again an hour before landing if your flight is so long that the first dose has worn off. Decongestants will help dry up the fluid in your sinuses and inner ears. But if you do take decongestants, make sure you drink extra fluids, because decongestants' dehydrating side effects, coupled with the already dry cabin air, will make your mouth, lips, and nose feel very dry. If your sinus problems are due to allergies, try a decongestant/antihistamine combination, available over-the-counter.

TRAIN, BUS, CAR

Traveling by automobile has one big comfort advantage over other means of transportation: the occupants control the vehicle. That means that you can plan your car trip for maximum comfort and minimum hassle.

The American Automobile Association advises that three hundred miles is the maximum amount of driving you should plan for a day. Stop the car every one hundred miles or so—or every two hours—to stretch your legs, walk around, and loosen stiff muscles. Make your lodging reservations in advance so you're never stuck looking for a place to stay when you're too tired to drive.

If you're taking a long trip by train or bus, consider making the journey in stages—with only a few hours of traveling each day, and a stopover every night in between. When long train or bus journeys must be completed in one stretch, follow the same rules for exercising as apply to jet travel. And while it's not necessary to avoid alcohol (unless you're driving!), caffeine, and soft drinks on the ground, try to eat lightly on the road to avoid sleepiness and/or motion sickness.

Finally, just because you are on vacation doesn't mean you can be lax about automobile safety rules. *Always* wear seatbelts. Make sure your children wear seatbelts, too, or are securely strapped into safety seats, depending on their ages. *Never* drive after drinking alcohol. And take special care on unfamiliar roads, in unfamiliar vehicles, and at night.

3 | Taking Your Stomach on the Road

Digestive problems are the most common travel complaint of all, and no wonder. Under the best of circumstances, your gastrointestinal routine is severely interrupted when you travel. Not only are you eating different foods than usual, in different amounts, and at different times, but you're doing it all under stress (strange conditions, unfamiliar language, and altered sleep, for example). In less than ideal conditions, the local food and water are likely to contain microorganisms hostile to your digestive tract. In fact, of the over two hundred countries in the world, less than one quarter have water safe for an American to drink. It's almost more surprising when people don't suffer tummy troubles than when they do.

The following is a guide to eating and drinking for good health, and a list of common "gut reactions"—how to prevent them, recognize them, and treat them.

The Facts about Foreign Food (and Drink)

The quick way to remember food and water safety is: "If you can't cook it, boil it, peel it . . . avoid it." Here are some specifics:

WATER

American intestines never come in contact with many of the micro-organisms common to underdeveloped countries. Our own chlorine-treated water has spoiled our gastrointestinal (GI) tracts so that they are unable to fight off foreign strains of bacteria. Our intestines are so unaccustomed to dealing with new organisms that Americans have even suffered from water-transmitted diarrhea when traveling from one part of the United States to another. For the same reason, an estimated 2 to 15 percent of foreign visitors to the United States also suffer from diarrhea. Besides common travelers' diarrhea, contaminated water can transmit such diseases as typhoid fever, cholera, polio, and hepatitis.

In general, the water of northern Europe, Great Britain, Australia, New Zealand, and Japan is safe for Americans to drink. The water of South and Central America, Asia, the Middle East, and Africa is usually not. In the Caribbean, the water quality varies. Some island water is fine for Americans, some not. You'll have to check with the local tourist board. In major cities around the world, large hotels that cater to tourists generally have safe, treated water: again, ask the management to be sure, but if you have doubts, take precautions anyway.

When the tap water isn't safe, stick to bottled or boiled water. Bring along an electric hot plate or an immersion coil with an adapter if you intend to boil your water. It should be boiled for ten minutes, then thoroughly cooled, before it is safe to drink.

Generally, carbonated bottled water is safer than plain bottled water both because carbonation seems to kill some microorganisms, and because dishonest hotel and restaurant personnel have been known to fill bottles with local tap water and recap them. Make sure the bottles have been properly sealed. (Check the mineral content of bottled water before drinking it if you are on a sodium-restricted diet.) To be extra careful, brush your teeth with bottled water, or even soft drinks, instead of tap water although some experts have suggested that brushing your teeth with local tap water is safe because most toothpastes contain antibacterial substances. If you decide to take your chances and use tap water to brush, be sure not to swallow any water when you rinse. (Don't swallow any water in the shower, either.)

Boiling is the best way to purify water yourself, since it kills all disease-causing organisms without affecting the water's taste. But when you're forced to drink local water and can't boil it—for instance, on hiking or backpacking trips—you should bring along water purifying tablets such as Halazone (a chlorine bleach) or Potable-Aqua (a buffered iodine agent), available in camping or sporting goods stores, and pharmacies. The tablets come with instructions for their use. Know that Potable-Aqua tablets lose their potency if left exposed to air, heat or moisture.

Alternately, you can purify water with ordinary chlorine liquid laundry bleach (4 to 6 percent) or tincture of iodine (2 percent). Mix five drops of iodine or two of bleach in a quart or liter of water. Let stand for half an hour. You should be able to taste the bleach or iodine faintly when you drink it. If you can't, add a little more and wait a while again. And if the water is cold or cloudy, use a double dose of iodine or chlorine, and then wait at least five hours before drinking. Strain cloudy water through a clean cloth before treating it. (Caution: Although it is rare, some people are sensitive to iodine and may develop a blotchy red skin rash after drinking water treated with it. Also, persons being treated for hyperthyroidism should not drink iodine-treated water.) Neither iodine nor chlorine is as effective a method of water purification as boiling.

Sporting goods and camping stores may carry mechanical filters for purifying water. These have the advantage of not affecting the water's taste; however, they are also not as effective as boiling water.

Beverages such as coffee and tea, prepared with boiling water and served hot, are safe to drink in restaurants. So are canned, undiluted fruit juices. Drinks that have been bottled and sterilized—such as beer, wine, and soft drinks—are also generally safe. But be wary of mixed drinks or drinks served with ice cubes—alcohol or freezing temperatures do not kill the microorganisms that can make you sick.

MILK AND DAIRY PRODUCTS

Avoid milk and dairy products (including cheeses, sauces made with milk or cream, ice cream and other desserts made with dairy products) in rural areas and developing countries where pasteurization is not as common as in the United States. Most English-speaking nations and developed countries require pasteurization by law. You can assume that if the water is not safe to drink, neither is the milk.

Unpasteurized, contaminated milk can transmit many diarrhea-causing intestinal infections, and such diseases as brucellosis (an illness with flu-like symptoms prevalent in southern Europe, Latin America, and central Asia, caused by a microorganism usually transmitted to humans via dairy products) and even tuberculosis.

Boil fresh, unpasteurized milk before drinking it. Canned, evaporated, condensed, or powdered milk is okay to drink if you dilute it with boiled, bottled, or purified water.

FOOD

In developing countries, stick mainly to cooked foods, and eat them while they're hot. Make sure all meat and poultry are thoroughly cooked, never rare.

Fish and shellfish must be eaten with caution. Shellfish, such as oysters, crabs, shrimp, and lobsters, can transmit cholera, typhoid, or hepatitis, as well as other gastrointestinal illnesses, unless they are very well cooked. Never eat raw oysters or clams. Even steaming is inadequate protection against illness. Eat sushi only in developed countries, in clean restaurants that cater to tourists, since raw fish can harbor a variety of parasitic worms.

Occasionally, even well-cooked fish can cause special types of food poisoning called scombroid or ciguatera fish poisoning. Seek medical attention if any of the following symptoms occurs within an hour of eating fish: diarrhea, muscle and joint pain, chills, sweating, nausea, vomiting, numbness, weakness, abdominal pain, paralysis, reversal of hot and cold sensation, dizziness, blurred vision or temporary blindness, itching, shock (all symptoms of ciguatera poisoning); or flushing, red facial rash, body rash, generalized itching, severe headache, dizziness, burning or numbness of the mouth and throat, shortness of breath, abdominal cramps, nausea, vomiting, diarrhea (all symptoms of scombroid fish poisoning).

Fruits and vegetables can be eaten in developing countries if they've been boiled, or can be peeled—by you—and not rinsed off in local water. Or scrub them with bottled water before eating them. Pass up any fruits or vegetables with broken skins or peels. Lettuce and salads are especially hazardous, since a multitude of parasites can live in the leaves.

Breads and baked goods are generally safe, as are most dry foods (unless hand-contaminated), because bacteria grow best on a moist surface. In underdeveloped countries, avoid picturesque markets and roadside stands; instead, frequent restaurants that have many travelers as patrons, and are more likely to follow the necessary hygiene precautions. Avoid smorgasbords and buffets, since the food is usually left out in the open for long periods. Ideally, you shouldn't even eat or drink from dishes that have been washed in local water. Don't be embarrassed about wiping dishes, glasses, and silverware with a napkin, or with an alcohol-soaked cleansing pad.

Don't ever take hygiene for granted—even the food and water on luxury cruise liners has been known to cause outbreaks of diarrhea and food poisoning on board. And don't relax your vigilance until you're safely home. The food, water, and ice you're served on board a plane returning to the States, for instance, can cause travelers' diarrhea because it is usually brought on board locally, not in America.

If you're concerned that these dietary restrictions will temporarily affect your nutrition, bring along a multivitamin supplement, and perhaps some bran tablets.

Travelers' Diarrhea

No matter what you call it—Montezuma's Revenge, the Aztec Two-Step, Delhi Belly, the Tokyo Trots, King Tut Gut, or simply "turista"—this common gastrointestinal ailment is the traveler's bane. In fact, there's an old saying: "Travel broadens the mind but loosens the bowel!" Despite the funny names and sayings, the condition is no joke; about one-third of its victims must take to bed, and another 40 percent must change their plans to accommodate the symptoms. An estimated one-third of Americans who travel to developing countries succumb to diarrhea; in Mexico, turista afflicts as many as half of all visitors from the States. Young adults are more likely to get travelers' diarrhea than older travelers, perhaps because they are more adventurous and daring about sampling the local cuisine, or perhaps because they have not yet developed immunity.

The causes of turista are varied. Most cases—an estimated 40 to 70 percent—are caused by a form of toxin-producing *Escherichia coli,* a bacteria that (in its benign form) is normally found in the digestive tract. But besides *E. coli* there are many other microorganisms—bacteria, viruses, and protozoa—that may also be responsible. These include *Vibrio parahaemolyticus, Shigella, Campylobacter jejuni, Salmonella,* Norwalk-like virus, rotaviruses, and *Giardia* (this last one a particular hazard to travelers in the Soviet Union). Usually, the organisms enter the body via food, drinking water, and ice cubes, but there are plenty of other transmission routes, including contaminated lakes, streams, and rivers in which tourists swim.

Following the safe food and water guidelines mentioned above is the best way to prevent turista, but the condition can be prevented with medications, too. These include Pepto-Bismol tablets, which are available over-the-counter, and prescription drugs like doxycycline, an antibiotic in the tetracycline family (brand name Vibramycin), and antimicrobial combination drugs that contain trimethoprim and sulfamethoxazole (brand names Bactrim and Septra).

Pepto-Bismol must be taken regularly to be effective. You will need to chew two tablets four times a day starting the day before you leave and continuing for two days after you return. Because Pepto-Bismol contains bismuth subsalicylate, which is an aspirin-like compound, persons who are sensitive or allergic to aspirin, have renal insufficiency, take anticoagulant therapy or are taking aspirin medications or medications that may interact badly with aspirin, should not take it. The main side effects of bismuth subsalicylate are blackening of the tongue and stool, which is disagreeable, but not harmful.

The prescription drugs each have advantages and disadvantages. They all carry the risk of side effects, including increased chance of certain fungal infections (such as vaginal yeast infections), sun sensitivity, and skin rashes. Occasionally, these drugs can even cause the diarrhea they were taken to prevent! Vibramycin has the advantage of helping to protect against chloroquine-resistant malaria as well as turista, but its disadvantage is that there are already strains of turista-causing organisms that have developed resistance to the drug in Mexico and other areas. Bactrim and Septra are more effective against *E. coli* and *Shigella,* and they can help prevent typhoid, too, but some people will discover they are allergic to the drugs.

Because travelers' diarrhea is usually more an uncomfortable condition than a dangerous one, a recent National Institutes of Health panel advised against using these drugs routinely as protection against turista. But if you have a special reason for wanting to remain well while away—because you're on a crucial business trip, for example, or on your honeymoon—you might want to consider them anyway. People who will be traveling to remote areas where food and water are not safe and medical facilities not easily available—such as those on a Himalayan trek or canoe trip down the Amazon—also have a valid reason for taking prophylactic drugs. So do elderly people, and those with certain medical conditions—coronary artery disease, diabetes, kidney disease—for whom a case of turista would be more serious than for most (see chapter 11). Also, people who take a lot of antacids or prescription drugs for ulcers should ask their doctors about prophylactic medication, since their altered stomach acidity may make turista more likely. Consult your physician for more information, and for a prescription.

If, in spite of all your precautions, turista strikes, it needn't ruin your trip. If you begin treatment for it immediately, you can usually get rid of the problem in a day and a half. Left untreated, most cases will go away by themselves in two to five days (although you may feel weak for several days afterward). Some doctors recommend not treating diarrhea unless it becomes serious, because diarrhea is actually the body's way of ridding itself of the invading organisms. But most travelers do not want to waste vacation or business time waiting for nature to take its course.

For a mild case of diarrhea (defined as one or two loose stools over an eight-hour period, accompanied by abdominal cramps, nausea, or malaise), you can take an antimotility drug such as loperamide (Imodium), or Pepto-Bismol. Imodium is a prescription drug; Pepto-

Bismol can be bought over-the-counter. Recent studies have confirmed the effectiveness of both these medications against travelers' diarrhea. Of the two, Imodium will relieve symptoms more quickly. Follow the instructions on the label. Some studies have shown that plain aspirin alone reduces stool volume. If you have nothing else available, it's worth a try.

For more serious cases (defined as three or four loose or watery bowel movements in an eight-hour period, accompanied by nausea, vomiting, abdominal cramps, or fever), it is truly time to take that antibiotic or antimicrobial drug. The medications used to treat turista—Bactrim, Septra, Vibramycin—are the same as those used to prevent it. Whether or not you intend to take these drugs in advance as protection against diarrhea, it makes sense to get yourself a prescription before you leave and take the medication with you just in case, so you won't have to buy medicine abroad. Some of the drugs available in other countries to treat diarrhea, such as Enterovioform and Mexaform (both of which contain iodochlorhydroxyquin), are not considered safe or effective by the U.S. Food and Drug Administration.

While you're battling turista, adjust your diet to lessen symptoms. Avoid solid foods, or at least eat lightly. Foods such as salted crackers, clear soups, dry toast or bread, gelatin, and sherbet are okay. Don't consume milk and dairy products, red meats, most fruits and vegetables, fatty or spicy foods, alcohol, or caffeine. As you start to feel better, you can begin to eat rice, baked potatoes, or chicken soup with rice or noodles. Then, as your symptoms continue to decrease, you can eat baked fish and poultry, applesauce and bananas. Within a week, you should be eating normally again.

But even more important than what you eat is what you drink, since if your diarrhea is severe, you run the risk of becoming dehydrated. Drink lots of bottled water, caffeine-free soft drinks, fruit juices, and broths. You can also drink Gatorade™ or use commercially available rehydration salts (called Gastrolyte) to prevent dehydration and replace electrolytes such as sodium and potassium. If you are urinating every four to five hours, it's a sign you're doing okay.

You can also prepare an effective rehydration concoction yourself:

In one glass: Mix 8 ounces of orange, apple, or other fruit juice rich in potassium, with ½ teaspoon of honey or corn syrup, and a pinch of table salt.

In a second glass: Mix 8 ounces of water (bottled, boiled, or purified) with ¼ teaspoon of baking soda.

Drink alternately from each glass until your thirst is quenched. And continue to drink plenty of other fluids as well. This formula should not be given to very young children (see chapter 10), or to adults with diabetes, heart or kidney disease, or adrenal gland disease.

If diarrhea persists beyond three days, or seems especially severe—for instance if the stool contains blood or is accompanied by severe abdominal pain—it's important to receive medical attention. You may not be suffering from run-of-the-mill travelers' diarrhea at all, but from something more serious.

For now, dietary caution and prompt treatment are the best ways to deal with "tummy bugs." But scientists are working on a vaccine against the condition, and travelers of the future may be able to visit their doctors for a shot before they depart, then throw caution to the wind and eat local fruits and vegetables to their hearts' delight anywhere in the world.

Constipation

Although it receives far less attention than diarrhea, constipation is actually very common among travelers. It's usually the result of a disruption in normal eating, drinking, sleeping, and exercising habits. Visitors to developed nations such as Japan, Northern Europe, or Australia, where turista is not a problem, may become constipated by this change in routine. Also, people who have eliminated fruits and vegetables from their diets in an attempt to avoid diarrhea in under-developed countries may suffer from constipation.

Try to keep your routine as close to what's normal for you as possible. While eating unfamiliar foods is part of the appeal of traveling, at least try to eat your meals at your usual time. (The next chapter offers tips on maintaining diet and fitness while traveling.) Drink lots of water (bottled if you're concerned about turista). The more water you drink, the more will reach your intestinal tract, where it's needed for elimination.

A diet rich in fiber (cereals and bran, fruits and vegetables) will also help alleviate the problem, so it may be worthwhile to bring along a box of bran or bran tablets or a can of prunes. If you often suffer from constipation, you may want to pack an over-the-counter bulk laxative such as Metamucil, a natural therapeutic fiber, to restore and maintain your regularity when traveling. While Metamucil can be used on an ongoing basis, other over-the-counter laxatives are safe for occasional use in relieving constipation.

Exercise can also help relieve constipation, and a brisk walk is good medicine. Just as a sedentary life-style can make your "outer body" flabby, a lack of exercise can make the muscles of the intestinal tract slow down, delaying bowel movements and causing constipation.

Constipation is usually nothing to be concerned about—in fact, many people who consider themselves chronically constipated are actually perfectly normal. Bathroom schedules are as individual as everything else about a person—some people have bowel movements three times a day; others three times a week. What's more important than how often you pass a stool, is how easily. As long as you are comfortable passing even a hard, dry stool, it doesn't matter whether you are passing it daily or not. Relax; most travelers' constipation will clear itself up in a few days once your body adjusts to the new routine.

It's time to seek medical attention for constipation if it occurs very suddenly, or if:

- it is accompanied by severe abdominal cramps and bloating;
- stools are very thin and pencil-like or ribbon-y;
- stools are pitch black, or you are passing blood (Note: Pepto-Bismol and other medications containing bismuth or iron can turn stools black, and in such a case there's no need to worry).

Stomachache Guide

Since you probably won't be choosing and preparing your own food, nor do you have the assurance of the local board of health that the food being put before you is safe, it's possible that something you eat while away from home won't agree with you. Travel conditions such as stress and fatigue may also bring on digestive difficulties—the connection between the mind and the stomach is a strong one. It's important to be able to discriminate among different kinds of abdominal pain, so you can treat common stomach problems effectively.

OVEREATING: THE "I CAN'T BELIEVE I ATE THE WHOLE THING" STOMACHACHE

This is probably the simplest stomach problem to treat, because the cause is so obvious. That second helping of pasta, the dessert you simply couldn't resist, or just the cumulative effect of morning 'til night nibbling, will manifest itself as an uncomfortable feeling of fullness and sluggishness. Time is the best healer for that stuffed feeling, but to ease your discomfort, rest for a few hours until some of the food has digested, and avoid tobacco, alcohol, and coffee—and more food—until you feel better. Eat lightly for at least twenty-four hours afterward.

INDIGESTION

Most people describe this condition as a feeling of food "not digesting right." For the traveler who is sampling exotic cuisines, or eating dinners late at night (as is fashionable in many Latin nations), indigestion is a common complaint. Over-the-counter antacids effectively relieve routine cases of indigestion, and can be taken several times a day as needed. The four most common types of over-the-counter antacids are sodium bicarbonate, calcium carbonate, magnesium salts, and aluminum. People with heart problems or high blood pressure should read the list of product ingredients carefully and avoid antacids containing bicarbonate of soda (baking soda); these antacids are high in salt. People on tetracycline medications should avoid antacids containing aluminum, calcium, or magnesium. Magnesium salt antacids can sometimes cause diarrhea, and aluminum salt antacids can cause constipation; the two ingredients are often combined in medication to offset each other's effect. Also, some "fizzy" antacids contain aspirin; avoid these products if you are allergic to aspirin, suffer from ulcers, or have a history of bleeding disorders.

HEARTBURN

Heartburn is so-called because the main symptom of the condition is a burning sensation in the lower chest. The burning feeling is caused by stomach acid backing up into the esophagus. Coughing, pregnancy, obesity, and constipation (because of straining to move the bowels) all aggravate this condition. Heartburn sufferers should stick to a bland diet, and avoid carbonated soft drinks, alcohol, caffeine, spicy foods, chocolate, and foods high in fat. If you're prone to heartburn, try to avoid exercising strenuously within two hours of eating; also avoid lying down, since a horizontal position increases the chances that the stomach's contents will move up into the esophagus. Wear clothing that is not tight or binding around the waist. To alleviate symptoms, taking an antacid is probably all that is necessary (use the cautions discussed in the section on Indigestion, above, to choose a product). If you frequently suffer from heartburn, however, you may have a hiatal hernia. This condition—in which a weakness in the diaphragm allows a small portion of the stomach to push into the chest cavity—is usually not serious (although a small number of cases do require surgery). But if symptoms persist, you should consult a physician to rule out other disorders.

GAS

Bloating, cramps, belching, and passing of flatus are the symptoms, and the causes range from swallowing air (eating too fast, chewing gum, smoking, drinking through a straw, sipping hot liquids, talking while eating), to consuming certain foods that the body finds difficult to digest (beans, peas, cabbage, cauliflower, broccoli, brussels sprouts, radishes, onions, and garlic, among others). Certain milk and grain products may result in gassiness in people whose systems are sensitive to these foods. Carbonated soft drinks are another common cause of gas. You can avoid gas by eliminating these foods from your diet, by eating more slowly, and by changing those habits that cause you to swallow air. Over-the-counter antiflatulants containing simethicone or activated charcoal may provide some relief.

FOOD POISONING

Spoiled food signals itself by its color, odor, or taste. Unfortunately, food contaminated with the various bacteria, toxins, and viruses that cause food poisoning generally looks and tastes fine. Travelers are at the mercy of the kitchen staff in every hotel, cruise ship, and restaurant they visit.

Generally, washing, refrigerating, and cooking at high temperatures are enough to kill these bacteria, but if food is left out at room temperature (or even kept warm on a stove) long enough, the bacteria may form a toxin that will survive subsequent heating or freezing. To be safe, in underdeveloped countries—or anywhere you don't trust the food and hygiene—avoid undercooked or raw meats, poultry, and fish. Don't order foods with cream sauces, homemade mayonnaise, or custards because they may spoil or become contaminated more quickly than other foods.

The majority of cases of food poisoning are not serious, and are caused by the *Salmonella, Staphylococcus aureus, Bacillus cereus,* and *Clostridium perfringens* bugs. These bacteria are not at all rare: They are present on the skin, in the intestines, in soil and dust, and in most unprocessed food.

The symptoms of food poisoning are similar to those of other common stomach disorders: abdominal pain, diarrhea, nausea, and vomiting. Fever may also occasionally be present. Depending on the specific toxin, the symptoms may appear anywhere from one hour to three days after eating contaminated food. And the symptoms will subside after six hours to a week, again depending on the specific poison. Bed rest and plenty of fluids (to prevent dehydration) is usually the recommended treatment for food poisoning. But medical attention may be required if symptoms include a high fever or bloody diarrhea, or if they last for more than a few days. In general, follow the instructions for treating travelers' diarrhea.

Another, much more serious, type of food poisoning is that caused by the organism *Clostridium botulinum*. And though rare, botulism poisoning is extremely dangerous, even deadly. The poison is usually found in foods in leaky or bulging cans, or in home canned goods. See a physician or head to an emergency room immediately if you experience any of these symptoms of botulism poisoning: difficulty in breathing, double vision, slurred speech, difficulty in swallowing, paralysis.

THE MIND/STOMACH CONNECTION

You probably know it as "nervous stomach," but doctors call it "irritable bowel syndrome." Rushing around, not sleeping enough, worrying about missing your plane, or forgetting something important, can all bring on symptoms of diarrhea, gas, indigestion, and lower abdominal pain, when there's no other cause than stress. To calm a nervous stomach, *relax*. Read an entertaining novel, take a warm bath, listen to soothing music on the hotel radio. Regular exercise also helps relieve symptoms. Try drinking warm water or eating saltine crackers or dry toast. An increase in dietary fiber—fruits, vegetables (well-cooked if you must be concerned about turista), and whole grains—can also lessen the symptoms for most people. A doctor can prescribe an antispasmodic medication to deal with recurrent bouts.

WHEN TO LOOK FOR A DOCTOR

If you've ruled out turista, overeating, heartburn, gas, food poisoning, and stress as the cause of your tummy troubles, you may need to seek medical attention. While the vast majority of stomach pains are no more than minor annoyances, sometimes they can signal a serious condition such as an ulcer, gallstones, colitis, or even cancer.

Consult a physician if you experience severe pain that lasts more than six hours, recurs more than three or four times, or is accompanied by shaking, chills, or cold, clammy skin. Also see a doctor if your stomachache is accompanied by any of the following: a fever that persists for more than two days or exceeds 101°F., unintentional weight loss or unexplained persistent appetite loss, prolonged upper abdominal bloating, persistent dizziness or fever, yellowish skin or tea-colored urine, blood in the vomit, pain or difficulty in swallowing food. A change in bowel habits that lasts for two weeks or more, or bowel movements containing blood, pus, or mucus, or stools that are black, tarry, gray, clay-colored, or pencil-thin also warrant medical attention.

Sometimes, the symptoms of heartburn or indigestion can feel frighteningly like a heart attack. Your own experience is your best guide to when a stomachache requires a visit to the doctor. Heart attack pain, which ranges from mild to excruciating, usually does not go away with rest, and lasts a half an hour or more. Sweating, nausea, vomiting, dizziness, or fainting may accompany the chest pain. Also, heart attack pain may radiate down an arm, or down the jaw or back; it may feel constricting or vise-like. If you are feeling a new kind of discomfort in your stomach or chest, one which doesn't feel like all the run-of-the-mill tummyaches you've had before, be on the safe side and go to an emergency room to rule out heart problems.

Most people consider eating the local foods an integral part of traveling. And it's hard not to resent restrictions on culinary adventurousness. But it's far better to observe the precautions and have the entire length of the trip to safely sample new foods, than to go "hog wild" at the outset of a voyage and spend several days nursing a traumatized digestive tract back into shape. *De gustibus!*

4 | Foreign Diet and Fitness

For most travelers, a vacation or business trip means a weight gain. Confronted with exotic cuisine served up in three big restaurant meals a day, many travelers throw up their hands in despair, open their mouths . . . and eat to their heart's content, blithely promising themselves to diet when they get home.

And food isn't the only reason for the weight gain. While some people may actually be getting more exercise—simply by walking— than usual, fitness fanatics with a regular routine usually leave their discipline behind when they travel. The combination of more food and less movement is a powerful—and fattening—one.

Obviously, it's not always possible to follow your regular diet and exercise program exactly when you're away. But with good judgment and common sense, you can travel home without excess baggage . . . in extra pounds.

Diet

Foreign food doesn't have to equal future fat. In fact, according to nutrition experts, there are many styles of cooking that are better for you than what you probably eat at home. In terms of calories and cholesterol, Mediterranean cuisine (especially southern Italian and Greek) and Asian food (especially Japanese) are considered the most healthful. The Mediterranean diet emphasizes olive oil (in moderation), fish and seafood, whole grain breads and pastas, and fresh fruits and vegetables—all nutritious, nonfattening, and low in cholesterol. The Japanese diet, while high in salt and preserved foods, stresses spartan meals of low-fat foods. If you're lucky enough to be traveling to one of these areas, eating like the natives could be the best thing for you.

Feast on pasta with cooked seafood, vegetables sautéed in a bit of olive oil, green salads, fresh fish, and rice. (Go easy, however, on the cheeses, heavy cream sauces, the Italian ice cream—called gelato—and Greek baklava.)

But if Asia or the Mediterranean isn't your destination, you'll have to try a little harder. First of all, plan ahead. When you reserve your hotel room, opt for the room alone without food included—you'll be less tempted to eat three large meals a day if you haven't already paid for them. If you're on a business trip with an expense account, avoid the temptation to order lots of food because your company is paying for it. Treat yourself to quality instead of quantity for more pleasure and fewer calories.

You may not be able to pack a bathroom scale, but you can still tell if you're putting on weight as you travel if you bring along a tape measure, and one pair of pants or a skirt that fits snugly. Try the tight item of clothing on every morning. When the buttons don't close and the zippers don't zip, you'll know you're in trouble. Alternately, bring along a belt and mark which notch fits at the start of your journey. Your waistline will be the first to show a weight gain.

Don't be embarrassed to bring along some of your own dietary supplies. For instance, low-calorie products are not available in much of the world. If you count on artificial sweetener for your morning coffee, the only way you'll be sure of having it is if you bring it along. A package of favorite hard candies might help you avoid fattening snacks—an enormously tempting vacation lure. Packages of rice cakes or melba toast, some dried fruit, and a jar of peanut butter could substitute for occasional breakfasts or lunches.

Just because you're away from home, don't forget the healthy eating habits you've been trying to cultivate for yourself. Why avoid butter all year, then smear tons of it on a croissant every morning for a week while you're away? If you avoid salt, sugar, and fats in your normal diet, traveling does not give you carte blanche to gorge yourself on fried foods and pastries, no matter how exotic and appealing they look.

Don't be embarrassed to make special requests at a restaurant or hotel. If you don't want a sauce on your fish, ask for it to be omitted. If you'd prefer that the bread not remain on the table, ask the waiter to remove it. After all, you're the paying customer and you have a right to enjoy things the way you like them.

If you are on a beach vacation, whether in the South Pacific, the Caribbean, or Florida, try to include foods rich in beta-carotene or Vitamin A in your diet. A recent study shows that sunlight destroys beta-carotene (which the body converts to Vitamin A) in the body, but that beta-carotene and Vitamin A actually protect against sunburn and some kinds of cancer (skin, lung, bladder, throat). Vitamin A also helps maintain healthy skin and hair, and is necessary for proper bone growth, tooth development, and reproduction. To avoid depleting your body of this essential nutrient while in the sun, eat plenty of beta-carotene- and Vitamin A-rich foods. These foods include: spinach, turnip greens, broccoli, squash, carrots, sweet potatoes, pumpkin, peas, cantaloupes, mango, papaya, brussels sprouts, cabbage, romaine lettuce, and parsley.

If you are traveling to a country noted for its spicy cuisine, such as Mexico, India, China, or the West Indies, know what to do if you accidentally bite into a fiery pepper: To extinguish the burning in your mouth, a glass of whole milk works better than water. Water can actually make the burning worse: Since the chemical in the spicy peppers that is responsible for the burn is not water-soluble, the water can distribute the burning sensation throughout your mouth. But the coldness of milk (or yogurt or sour cream) will help stop the burn, while the milk fat coats the mouth and relieves pain. Acidic drinks, and beverages with oil, or alcohol can help, too, since they can mix with the hot chili oils and reduce the chemical reaction that causes the burn; try tomato juice or lemonade. And sugary or starchy foods—such as pasta, bread, rice, or potatoes—can also help absorb some of the peppers' heat.

Savoring the local cuisine may be part of the travel adventure, but every country and culture has its healthy foods as well as its unhealthy ones, and eating the right foods still counts as a cultural experience. Locally grown fruits and vegetables (provided turista isn't a problem) are as much a part of the local diet as locally baked breads and cakes. A region's mineral water is as representative of it as its wines. (Check the label carefully for the sodium content if you are on a restricted diet.)

Learn to focus less on the food itself, and more on the rituals that accompany serving and eating food. Notice the restaurant's decor, the attentiveness of the waiters, the presentation of the food on the plate. And you don't always have to eat in your hotel or even in restaurants. Buy foods such as breads, fruits, and cheeses to pack for a picnic.

Make up your mind that you will not eat three large meals each day. You can try one of several strategies. First, try eating as many Europeans do: a light breakfast usually consisting of bread or a roll and coffee, tea, or hot chocolate; a large lunch that is similar to an American supper, generally including meat, fish or chicken, and a vegetable; and a light evening meal of soup or salad. Calories consumed early in the day are more easily burned by the body than those consumed closer to bedtime.

Or you can try eating two meals instead of three. Combine your meals American-style by eating brunch in the late morning and dinner at the usual time. Or combine your meals British-style and eat a large breakfast at your usual time and then high tea in the late afternoon. Either way, you're eliminating one entire meal without leaving yourself open to hunger. If you must eat three meals, try allowing yourself to indulge in gourmet dinners, but eat lightly at breakfast and lunch. Whatever you do, avoid snacking.

If you're on a cruise, some of these choices won't be available to you—after all, you can't leave the ship to search for a restaurant with a fresher salad or plain broiled fish, or find a market to pack yourself a picnic. With their groaning tables laden with buffets of luscious food constantly available and already paid for, cruises are a dieter's nightmare. Try to offset the damage by limiting yourself to one dessert, one piece of bread, one glass of wine daily. Sample small portions of several different foods instead of taking large servings of each. Never allow yourself to go back for seconds at a buffet table. But most important, focus on the ship's activities, not on the food. Leave the ship each time it docks and take a walking tour. Swim, sign up for exercise classes, even play shuffleboard if it will pull you away from the dining hall or the poolside buffet table. It may not be easy, but it can be done.

One of the biggest reasons people gain weight while traveling is alcohol, which is fattening in quantity. It's almost inevitable that you will drink while away, but try not to drink at every meal . . . or with every course. Sip one glass of exquisite wine, lift a mug of local ale . . . but don't order a second round. Experiment with local mineral water as an alternative.

All this advice may sound daunting, but it's not as tough as it seems. As more and more people become health-conscious, hotels and restaurants are trying to accommodate travelers by offering lighter fare. Light cuisine is becoming more popular around the world. After all, even France, known for its rich sauces and luscious patisseries, was the originator of nouvelle cuisine, a sort of gourmet diet food. Many hotels and restaurants now offer two menus—one for the gourmand who wants to try it all, regardless of calories, and one for those determined to return home exactly the same weight as when they left.

One last note on food: People following special diets—those with medical conditions such as high blood pressure or diabetes, for example, or those with religious strictures (Orthodox Jews, Mormons, Moslems, Hindus, etc.)—will have to be especially careful, and especially resourceful. Wire ahead to your hotel to inform them of your dietary needs; most will do their best to accommodate you. Bring along packaged foods to tide you over when you can't find something suitable on the menu. Learn how to ask in a foreign language for what you need.

Fitness

Fitness is as much a matter of attitude as exercise. There are elevators and there are staircases; which one you take depends on your attitude. You can take buses, subways, and taxis . . . or you can bicycle or walk. Walking, especially, is one of the best exercises there is, and there's no excuse for avoiding it whether you're away on business or pleasure.

The benefits of exercise go beyond weight control. Regular exercise can actually reduce travel stress and fatigue, help deal with the symptoms of jet lag (if you exercise at the same time as you do at home), and help prevent constipation. Try to set aside about thirty minutes each day for exercise; dividing it between stretching and aerobics is ideal. You can even combine activities for more efficiency. For instance, make your fifteen minutes of aerobics a brisk walk from one place to another, instead of taking a cab.

With a little research and creativity, any traveler can make sure he or she stays fit. Obviously, if you've gone off on a ski vacation, or to a golf or tennis resort, you needn't worry about inactivity. But those whose travel time is crammed with business meetings, or full of days spent lazing in the sun, will need to take action.

If you're headed for a beach vacation, turn it to your favor. *Swim*, don't just wade or loll around in the water. Set a goal for distance, and try to go a bit further each day. Instead of simply parking your body on a towel and facing the sun, take long walks looking for seashells, try a new sport such as waterskiing, sailing, snorkeling, or scuba diving. Do anything rather than lie there drinking piña coladas.

Take advantage of every fitness service available to travelers. Many hotels, especially in Europe, have spas, gyms, or gym equipment. Cruise ships run exercise classes and have gym rooms; even some airports offer sports and exercise facilities for travelers with time to kill between flights. Ask the hotel concierge to recommend a safe jogging route, or to direct you to a local spa or gym. If you have a health club membership at home, you may be eligible for guest privileges in other clubs, even abroad. Other hotels offer guest privileges at local health clubs to their own guests.

Turn any hotel room or cruise ship cabin into a mini-gym. If you'll be missing regular aerobics classes while you're away, bring along a jump rope for an easy-to-cart-along aerobic workout. If you take a workout class at home, take along a Walkman℗ and some exercise cassettes— no one will hear your routine. (You can even ask your exercise instructor for permission to tape a class before you go away; that way you'll have your regular routine with you when you travel.)

Other easily-portable equipment: New rubber band and rubber tubing exercise gear that use the tension of the cable or band to increase the resistance to your muscles while you exercise. Light plastic or inflatable travel weights that can be packed empty (and weigh nearly nothing), and filled when you reach your destination. Fill them with water, which weighs about half a pound per cupful, for an easier routine; fill them with sand, which weighs about a pound per cupful, for a more strenuous workout. You can also use empty plastic soda or mineral water bottles, filled with water or sand, as handweights. A 1-liter bottle, filled with water, will weigh a little over two pounds.

Whatever you choose to do, be sure to begin exercising at a lower intensity than usual on a trip. Traveling, with its time changes, dietary changes, and stress, is draining. Start by running a shorter distance, doing fewer repetitions of calisthenics such as sit-ups, lifting lighter weights. Work up to your regular exercise program slowly—allow about one day per time zone crossed to build up to your regular routine.

Take the environment into account, and your own condition (for more information, see chapter 6 on the environment, and chapter 7 on sports savvy). Travelers who have left a cold climate for a hot one should really take it easy—the body actually needs several weeks to become fully acclimatized to heat. Going from a low altitude to a high one (above five thousand feet) also demands that you begin exercise slowly and gradually work up to your regular routine. Don't exercise for at least a day following your arrival so that your body can adjust to the new air pressure and oxygen level. If breathing seems difficult or your heart starts pounding rapidly, *stop* your workout.

No matter what the environment, make sure you drink plenty of water to replenish what you lose by being active. Cold water is better than warm, and uncarbonated water is better than carbonated. Don't wait until you feel thirsty to drink, either. The body doesn't register thirst until you've lost up to four pounds of fluid. To avoid dehydration, drink a glass of water before exercise, take water breaks every fifteen minutes or so, then drink a glass or two again after exercise.

While you're away, your goal shouldn't be to increase your fitness level, but merely to maintain it. Experts say that it takes a week to ten days before your fitness starts diminishing. That means that on a short trip, you needn't feel obligated to push yourself to the limit. For fitness fanatics, a week off every four months or so may actually be good for the body. For people who lead fairly sedentary lives, however, a vacation is a good opportunity to become a bit more active by walking a lot or swimming, for example. (Check with a physician before beginning an exercise program if you're over thirty-five.)

Fitness in a new environment requires a lot of common sense. Don't exercise alone, especially if you're jogging along unfamiliar streets. A partner provides some safety in less secure neighborhoods. Wear or carry identification when you exercise; in case of a medical emergency, it will be able to speak for you when you can't. One particularly good form of identification for exercisers is the Alert-Along Medical I.D. Tag. The plastic tag can be worn around the neck or tucked into sneaker laces. It's even backed with a light-reflecting strip to protect against nighttime accidents. The tag costs $2 (or you can get three for $5). Write to: Alert-Along Medical I.D. Tag, The Weiss Works, P.O. Box 374, Elkhart, IN 46515. Or call: (219) 294-2790.

Finally, never force yourself to exercise if your body is telling you that the stress of travel is simply too much for it at the moment. Instead, relax with a massage or hot bath to soothe muscles and mind.

5 | Body Parts That Need Tender Loving Care

Your Feet

When deskbound travelers head for adventure abroad, leaving behind their automobiles and their intimate knowledge of local mass transit systems, the feet are one of the first things to suffer. Aching, sore, tired, blistered feet are enough to make anyone want to forget exploring and head back for the hotel room. But there are both preventive and therapeutic measures for the feet.

First of all, it's important to pack proper footwear. Pointy-toed boots for men and stiletto-heeled pumps for women may be all the rage, but they won't carry anyone from one end of the Champs Elysées to another, much less down a cobblestone street or a country path. Bring along impractical fashion footwear if you must, but only for special evenings out—when a taxi will take you from hotel to restaurant to theater and home again.

But it's not necessary to go to the other extreme, either. Women needn't clomp around in bulky running shoes or men in clunky hiking boots to be comfortable. Invest in a compromise pair of shoes before you go. For women, a low (no more than an inch and a half) and not too narrow-heeled pair of shoes in a soft leather or comfortable canvas (both stretch), with a cushioned sole and plenty of room in the toes, is the best bet. Women should also avoid binding socks, pantyhose, or stockings, which can cut circulation, and older women should consider wearing a light elastic or support pantyhose. For men, a soft pair of leather or canvas shoes with flexible crepe or rubber soles will be most comfortable.

If you plan to be doing much of your city sightseeing in casual jeans or slacks, both men and women *are* probably best off in a good pair of sneakers with plenty of cushioning and support. Jogging or running sneakers are also good for walking. These shoes provide heel support (look for at least a quarter of an inch higher than the outer sole), shock absorption (padded soles), and stability (wide heels). Make sure the shoe fits properly, with half an inch of space between your longest toe and the shoe; there should be at least three eyelets for lacing, and the shoe should hold your heel firmly in place. Beware tennis sneakers, aerobics sneakers, basketball sneakers, etc. These sneakers were not made with the proper support or cushioning for long-distance walking, and are best left on the exercise mat, tennis court, or playing field. Don't go barefoot—parasites can enter the body through the soles of the feet.

Many shoe manufacturers are now making special walking shoes for men and women that are an attractive alternative to sneakers. Americans may be accustomed to the sight of well-dressed women walking to work in elegant business suits or skirts with sneakers and sweat socks, but the rest of the world is still catching on.

Whatever shoes you bring, make sure you bring along several pairs that you consider comfortable. If you develop blisters or other aches from one pair, switching to another will usually help relieve the pain, since different shoes put pressure on different parts of the foot.

Next, and just as important as having the proper footwear, is giving yourself plenty of time before your trip to break in your shoes . . . and your feet. If you're going to buy new shoes for traveling, try to purchase them at least a month before you leave so you can get accustomed to wearing them. Start taking walks every day for a couple of weeks before you leave, each day increasing the distance slightly. Wear the shoes you intend to take with you. You can prevent sore feet and leg cramps by building up your walking endurance slowly.

Besides walking, you can do exercises to prepare your feet for your trip. Sit in a straight-backed chair, and alternately point and flex your bare toes, first by themselves, then using your hands to bend your toes as far up and as far down as you can. Rotate your ankle in one direction, then the other. Press the soles of your feet together as hard as you can. Paint imaginary pictures or write invisible messages on the floor with your big toes. Try to pick up a (real) pencil with your toes.

Stand up and continue your exercises. Raise yourself on your toes for a count of twenty-five, several times a day. Starting with your feet flat on the floor, roll each foot outward twenty times, pressing the outer side to the floor. Then, with one foot on the floor, bend the other foot back and raise the toes toward your body as far as you can. Repeat with the other foot.

These exercises will strengthen muscles and joints, and help prevent sore feet and tired legs. You wouldn't run a marathon without training for it far in advance, so why demand extra walking endurance from your legs and feet without preparing properly? For extra effectiveness, you should continue to do these exercises while you're away.

If in spite of these precautions you wind up with foot fatigue or other problems, you can do a lot to ease the discomfort. Try one of the following recipes for a quick feet pick-me-up:

1). For instant relief, roll your foot back and forth over a cold soda or beer can. The combination of the cold and the rolling massage will make feet feel better in no time.

2). For a more complete treatment, soak your feet in cool salt water for ten minutes. Use one cup of Epsom salts per one gallon of water. (You should be able to find Epsom salts in a local pharmacy. If you're on a beach vacation, just use the ocean instead.) Dry your feet thoroughly, then give your feet and calves a massage with an oil, cream, or lotion. Some cosmetics companies make special foot creams containing such ingredients as cocoa butter or lanolin to soften hard skin, peppermint oil to combat odor, and menthol for an invigorating tingle. If you don't have a special foot cream, a hand cream containing urea (to soften skin) will work almost as well. Elevate your feet (above hip level) for five minutes.

3). For a thorough, and absolutely heavenly, foot massage, place one washcloth under cold water, and one under hot water. Then, alternating between them, give yourself a massage, starting with the arch of your foot and your calves. Place one hand at the big toe joint and the other at the fifth toe joint and start rubbing at half-inch intervals along the inside and outside of your foot. When you get to the ankle, put your fingertips on the front of your leg and your thumbs on the back and alternately squeeze every half inch all the way up to the knee, and then back down. You're ready to pound the pavement again!

Beyond plain old sore feet, more specific foot problems—foot cramps, blisters, corns, calluses, athlete's foot, ingrown toenails—are equally treatable. (Diabetics and people with circulatory problems should check with their physician before attempting any kind of foot self-care, or even massage.)

Foot cramps are muscle spasms caused by fatigue, and by extra strain on one part of the foot due to improper walking habits (such as a lopsided gait) or taking up a new sport. The cramps occur very suddenly, often while you're sleeping or relaxing. To ease the cramp, massage your foot, and try to stand on a cold surface or wrap your foot in a cold towel. If you're plagued by frequent, painful cramps, see a physician.

Blisters are caused by friction, pressure against the skin that causes the top layer to separate from the skin below. The space in between fills with fluid. The best way to treat blisters is not to pop them, but to bandage them, ideally with a doughnut-shaped corn or bunion pad. The blister will usually heal itself. If the blister pops, press against it with a piece of sterile gauze to drain the fluid. (Some people can't resist popping blisters themselves. If you're one of them, at least do it safely. Sterilize a needle with alcohol or a match. Puncture the blister from the side, and then gently push out the fluid, pressing against it with a piece of sterile gauze.) Make sure you leave the top flap of skin in place; it protects against infection and speeds healing. Then, apply a topical antibiotic cream to the blister, and cover it with a Band-Aid™ or gauze pad. See a doctor if infection sets in.

Corns and calluses are also caused by friction, generally by poorly fitting shoes rubbing against the foot. A broad area of prolonged friction results in a callus, a very small area results in a corn. Calluses can also form because of unequal weight distribution. For instance, a woman who usually wears high heels may develop calluses on the balls of her feet from the constant pressure. Obviously, the best way to treat corns and calluses is to stop wearing the shoes that cause the problem. But away from home, your selection of footwear may be limited (as is your access to a competent podiatrist or orthopedic surgeon), and more temporary relief is required. Use a pumice stone to remove the top layer of rough skin gently from the corn or callus. (Do not use medicated disks or paint-on corn removers—these contain acid and can irritate the skin. Don't attempt do-it-yourself surgery either, or you may wind up with an infection far more painful than your original problem.) Finish by using a moisturizing or softening lotion. For a callus, which is usually not painful, this gentle abrasion is all the treatment that's called for until you get home and decide whether or not to see a foot specialist. For a corn, cover the area with a doughnut-shaped piece of moleskin or other soft material after you've used the pumice stone, to protect the corn from further irritation. These measures should allow you to finish your trip in comfort. You can see a doctor when you get home for more permanent relief.

Athlete's foot is a common fungal infection that may strike travelers unaccustomed to a lot of walking (and foot perspiration). More than twenty species of fungus may be responsible for this condition. The most common form of athlete's foot is an itchy, moist infection between the toes, and the best way to prevent it is also one of the best ways to treat it: Keep your feet very dry. Wash and dry your feet thoroughly every day, especially between the toes, and use powder afterward. (Don't use cornstarch, since it actually encourages the growth of fungal organisms.) Wear shoes that allow for ventilation, like sandals, or shoes made of natural materials such as leather and canvas, which allow feet to breathe. Cotton, rather than nylon, socks are best. If keeping your feet dry isn't sufficient, use an antifungal cream, ointment, or powder (the most effective contain tolnaftate) between your toes each day. If your feet don't respond to this treatment in a week or so, or if the athlete's foot spreads beyond the web space between your toes to the soles or sides of your feet, see a doctor for more powerful treatment.

Ingrown toenails can be prevented by avoiding shoes that press on the toenails, and by keeping the toenails clipped straight across, with the corners just *slightly* filed with an emery board to remove sharp edges and prevent the nail from penetrating the skin. Once an infection occurs—characterized by redness and swelling—avoid the urge to try and clip the nail. Instead, soak your foot for ten minutes, twice a day, in warm, salted water. Dry the foot carefully, then place a tiny bit of absorbent cotton between the skin and the corner of the nail (you may need a nail file, tweezer, or toothpick to do this). If the infection persists for more than three days, see a physician or podiatrist.

Your Back

Heavy suitcases, long periods of sitting on a plane, train, or bus, and sometimes overly soft foreign mattresses can all take their toll on your back. As usual, it's up to you, the traveler, to take a tough situation and make it work.

PACKING RIGHT   Third World natives who carry heavy loads on their heads have the right idea, as do modern-day bohemians with backpacks. But for most of the rest of us, trunks, suitcases, garment bags, and carry-on cases are a fact of the traveling life. And while carrying heavy suitcases may be good exercise for Arnold Schwarzenegger, it's not likely to do the rest of us much good, and it may do our backs a lot of harm. The best thing for your back is to invest in a luggage cart, or a suitcase with attached wheels and a strap for pulling (although pushing is even better for your back). If neither of these is possible, try to pack your things so that the weight is equally balanced between two bags. In other words, instead of one enormous suitcase and a light carry-on bag, pack your belongings in two medium-sized bags. You can also carry a bag with a shoulder strap bandolier-style, across your chest; switch sides every fifteen or twenty minutes. When you pick up your luggage, bend at the knees, not at the waist, so that you are lifting with your legs, rather than your back. Your back should remain straight. Perhaps most important of all for bad-back sufferers: Call a porter or bellhop whenever possible!

PROPER POSTURE   When you have to spend hours in a cramped airline seat, or on a bumpy bus or train ride, your back may ache in protest. But learning how to sit properly can help prevent these aches and pains. First of all, try to sit in a straight-backed chair with a firm cushion; slouching in a seat with your legs stretched out increases pressure on back disks and ligaments. If you can't find a suitable seat, placing a pillow behind your lower back will help. Keep your knees bent while sitting; ideally, they should be about an inch higher than your hips (you may need a small footstool, piece of luggage, or a stack of books and magazines under your feet to achieve this). Don't sit with your legs crossed, since it reduces circulation. Don't slump your shoulders, arch your back, or extend your stomach. Straight, correct posture helps keep your spine aligned and your back muscles strong.

Don't sit for long distances without taking any breaks. You should get up as often as possible to walk around a bit and stretch the muscles of your neck, back, and legs. When you rise from your seat for your break, it's best for your back if you slide your body off the seat first, rather than leading with your shoulders.

R_x FOR FLIMSY MATTRESSES   You may not consider a fluffy European featherbed or squishy foam rubber mattress a luxury when you're accustomed to a firm mattress at home. In this situation, you have only a few options:

1). Ask your hotel if they have other mattresses available, or if not, perhaps a cot with a firmer mattress.

2). See if you can find a wooden board to slip between the bed frame and the mattress to give your back more support.

3). If all else fails and you can't bear the thought of sleeping on such a soft bed, pile the mattress and linens on the floor and sleep there.

The best positions for sleeping, according to back experts, are either lying on your side and drawing one or both knees up toward your chin (the "fetal" position), or lying on your back with a small pillow under your knees to keep your back straight.

While it may be hard to believe, you can help your aching back by supporting your feet. If you suffer from nagging low backaches, you can relieve your pain by placing foot arch supports—the kind found in any drugstore—in your shoes. The supports act as shock absorbers to the body's muscles and bones. They reduce the jolt that occurs each time the heel strikes the ground when you're walking or running.

Other methods for relieving back pain are analgesics (aspirin, acetaminophen, ibuprofen, etc.), ointments (such as Ben-Gay) for sore muscles, hot baths and heating pads (or even a towel run under hot water), ice packs, or bed rest (when necessary). Many people who suffer from chronic back pain have been helped by regular exercise, which strengthens the back and stomach muscles. While a vacation or business trip is not the time to begin such a program, it may be worthwhile asking your doctor or checking with your local YMCA (Y's across the country are offering a course called "The Y's Way to a Healthy Back") for specifics either before your trip, or after you return.

Your Skin

Taking winter-pale skin into the sun, already dry skin into the desert, or acne-prone skin into a hot, humid climate can be a disaster. An artificial, instant seasonal change—winter to summer in one day, for instance, when you fly from New York to Jamaica in December—can take its toll on unprepared skin. Travelers must learn how to alter their usual skin care routines to cope with such factors as sun, heat, humidity, cold, dryness, salt water, chlorine, dust, smog, and pollution.

Here are tips on how to cope with the major environmental threats to your skin's health:

THE SUN

Unprotected sun exposure poses the greatest danger to your skin. Besides being the single largest risk factor for skin cancer, the sun (in addition to heredity and such lifestyle factors as smoking and drinking habits) is responsible for how quickly your skin ages. Whether you've gone on vacation specifically for a winter dose of sunshine, are spending your summer weekends at the beach, will be skiing down snowy slopes, or simply plan to be outdoors hiking, walking, or sightseeing, you should always shield your skin from the sun's rays. Remember that the sun's harmful effects—from wrinkles to cancer—are usually the cumulative result of many years of unprotected exposure.

People with light skin, eyes, and hair color, and those who have a history of burning easily, are most at risk for skin cancer, but doctors stress that *everyone* should take precautions. There are a bewildering array of products on the market for just this purpose, and choosing among them can be confusing. *Suntan lotions or oils* offer little or no protection against the sun, and are designed specifically to help people tan. Almost all dermatologists recommend that people avoid these products in favor of a sunscreen or sunblock. *Sunscreens* contain chemicals to help filter out harmful ultraviolet rays. They are labeled according to their SPF, or sun protection factor. An SPF of 4, for example, would allow you to stay in the sun for four times longer than usual without burning. The higher the SPF number, the more ultraviolet rays are screened by the product. An SPF of 15 is designed to filter out all ultraviolet light. *Sunblocks,* such as zinc oxide, block the sun by placing an opaque barrier between it and your skin. Though sunblocks are effective, most people prefer to use sunscreens, which are transparent, and do not show on the skin. Most dermatologists, who now believe that any but the most minimal sun exposure is harmful to the skin, recommend that people use strong sunscreens with an SPF of 15 or higher for near total protection against the sun.

Whether you choose a cream, lotion, or gel preparation is a matter of personal preference, but if you have problems with acne, a heavy cream or lotion could clog your pores and cause breakouts. To avoid them, look for an oil-free sunscreen with a light alcohol base. And don't forego the protection because you've noticed the sun helps clear up your acne; you'll experience some of the same benefits through a sunscreen, and protect your skin from burning at the same time.

If you persist in believing that a suntan is healthy-looking in spite of medical knowledge that it damages your skin, at least go about tanning prudently. The sun is strongest, and you are most likely to burn, between 10 A.M. and 2 P.M., so you should avoid sunning yourself during these hours. It's also possible to burn while wearing a thin or wet T-shirt, while sitting under an umbrella or palm tree (because the sand reflects the rays), while swimming, and even on an overcast day, so protect yourself accordingly. Start with a strong sunscreen or sunblock, and very gradually increase your time in the sun. If you intend to switch to products with a lower SPF number, do so very gradually and carefully to avoid burning. Follow the package directions about applying sunscreens; most advise that you first apply them twenty minutes to an hour before sun exposure, and then reapply them every few hours, or after swimming. Always apply them generously.

Sunscreens and sunblocks are not only for those whose major pastime is sunbathing. These products are intended for anyone who will be spending time outdoors. City sightseeing, usually done on foot, exposes you to more sun than you realize. Sailors and golfers certainly need protection. Skiers are particularly at risk, both because snow reflects the sun's rays, and because the high altitude means the sun is even stronger than at sea level (there is less atmosphere at higher altitudes to filter the ultraviolet rays). Many women's cosmetics manufacturers now produce moisturizers and foundations containing sunscreens. These products are ideal for the casual kind of sun exposure that occurs during most sightseeing.

The face is not the only part of your body that needs protection from the sun. The feet, stomach, thighs, and back, all of which are usually covered by clothing, are especially sensitive to sun exposure. Keep these areas covered when you're not swimming, or use a high SPF product. When you apply sun protection, make sure to extend the cream or lotion underneath your bathing suit, so that you won't burn if the edges slip. Other sensitive areas that may need special protection: lips, nose, underarms, the backs of the knees, and the hands (which, like faces, are almost constantly exposed, and subsequently age more quickly than other parts of the body). Cover the top of your head with a bandanna or hat unless your hair is especially thick and doesn't have an unprotected part—even scalps can burn. Finally, women who expect to spend time in the sun should be careful about wearing perfume. Many fragrances will react with sunlight to cause a rash or discoloration on the skin. It's best to save perfume for evening or indoor occasions.

HEAT

When your environment is hot and dry, your main concern should be drinking plenty of fluids to keep your whole body, including your skin, sufficiently hydrated. Moisturize your skin often, especially if you shower or swim frequently.

When heat is combined with humidity, however, increased perspiration and oiliness can cause clogged pores, acne breakouts, jock itch, and prickly heat rashes on areas of the body where skin rubs against skin (under the arms, between the legs, underneath the breasts). In this instance, you must try to keep the skin as clean and dry as possible. Loose clothing made of natural fibers such as cotton and linen will allow air to circulate and perspiration to evaporate. Wash skin frequently, and use an alcohol-based astringent on areas that are especially oily. Extend your cleansing routine beyond your face, to other areas of the body which will be bared in the hot weather, or that are also acne-prone (back, shoulders, chest). Use powder on your body after showering, especially on the friction-prone areas mentioned above. For jock itch, use antifungal powders—you can usually use the same brand of powder you use for athlete's foot (check the label). And women who continue to use a moisturizer in spite of high humidity should at least switch to a lighter, less oily product, and apply it only to those areas that truly need more moisture, like the skin around the eyes. (When you come inside, however, especially if you come in from a hot, humid environment into a very dry, air-conditioned building, you should give your skin the benefit of some extra moisture by applying body lotion, hand cream, facial moisturizer.)

COLD

Cold and dry seem to go together like hot and humid. And the biggest problem this duo causes is dry, itchy, chapped skin, a common problem in winter, or on ski vacations. Dermatologists even have a name for this condition: xerosis.

The solution is moisture, in the form of lip balm, body lotion, facial moisturizers, hair conditioners, etc. And while long, hot showers may appeal after a day in the cold, they do *not* help soothe dry winter skin, and can in fact make dryness and itching worse. Too-frequent bathing continually removes the natural, protective layer of oil from your skin's surface. Also, hot water opens the skin's pores and allows moisture to evaporate.

In the winter, take shorter, warm (rather than hot) showers. Switch from your summer deodorant soap to a mild "superfatted" or pH-balanced soap or a non-soap cleanser. Avoid alcohol-based products. Pat your skin dry rather than rubbing it vigorously. After you bathe, while the skin is still damp, apply a moisturizing lotion or oil. Use extra protection on your hands, face (especially around the eyes), and lips. If you're going to be outdoors for any period of time in harsh weather, wear protective clothing such as a scarf, gloves, even a ski mask. Ideally—but unfortunately not always possible when you're away from home—you should use a humidifier indoors, or place a pan of water by the radiator.

You may also need to protect delicate nasal membranes. Cold, dry weather can cause blood vessels to crack, resulting in nosebleeds. You can lubricate the inside of your nostrils—especially the septum (the dividing structure in the middle of your nose)—with a mild lubricating ointment such as Vaseline or Borofax, or with a soothing lotion of rosewater and glycerine, applied with your finger, or with a cotton swab.

Other threats to clear, glowing skin:

SALT WATER AND CHLORINE Two more elements that rob skin of moisture. After swimming in either one, rinse off with plain water, then apply a moisturizer. Protect your hair by rinsing and conditioning after swimming.

DUST, SMOG, POLLUTION   A trip to Tokyo, Los Angeles, or New York could expose your skin to more plain old dirt than usual. Avoid breakouts by stepping up your cleansing routine: wash your face several times a day rather than just in the morning and at night, and perhaps use a stronger soap or cleanser than usual (as long as you don't dry out your skin). For women, wearing makeup and foundation can actually protect the skin against dirt and pollution, since the makeup is a clean barrier between the dirty environment and the skin.

Your Eyes

The sun is as potent an enemy to your eyes as it is to your skin. Whether on a tropical isle or a sparkling ski slope, the sun's rays have the power to do your eyes a great deal of harm. Recent studies have suggested that repeated exposure to the sun's ultraviolet light (the invisible light responsible for tanning and burning) may eventually cause the type of cataracts commonly associated with aging. Other potential harm from the sun includes corneal and retinal damage, and cancer of the eye and eyelid.

The right sunglasses can screen out this light and protect the eyes. (Added benefits: the glasses protect the eyes from dust and wind, and they also help prevent wrinkles, since you won't squint when you wear them.) One of the best investments you can make in your eyes' future is to buy a good pair of sunglasses with lenses that effectively screen out ultraviolet rays. And while anyone who is spending time outdoors should wear these glasses, people with light-colored eyes, those who wear contact lenses, and people who have recently had eye surgery are especially sensitive to sunlight. (Birth control pills, certain diuretic drugs used to control high blood pressure, tranquilizers, anti-acne drugs like tetracycline and sulfa-based drugs can also increase the eyes'—and the body's—sensitivity to sun.)

Before you buy sunglasses, you should know what to look for in a lens—both the material and the color make a difference (the same holds true for regular and prescription lenses). Recent studies have found that in general, plastic lenses are more effective than glass, and green and gray tints are better than rose, blue, or yellow-colored lenses. Green and gray are best both because of their light-screening capabilities and because they tend to distort vision the least. Your lenses should be dark enough so that someone can't see your eyes clearly through them.

There are no hard and fast rules about lens darkness, color, or material, however, and even a very dark lens may not adequately screen out ultraviolet rays. In fact, a dark lens that *doesn't* screen out UV rays can do your eyes more harm than good. Your pupils will dilate in response to the dark . . . and more of the invisible UV light will reach your retinas and corneas. Look for lenses labeled as meeting the voluntary requirements of the American National Standards Institute, which specify that over 99 percent of ultraviolet B light must be screened out for a pair of glasses to be considered ultraviolet filters. *Any* glasses that claim to screen ultraviolet rays should have a tag stating the amount of UV rays they absorb. If there's no tag, you can ask the retailer or the manufacturer for the information: It should be listed in the manufacturer's catalogue. Polarized lenses help cut down on glare, but have nothing to do with screening out ultraviolet light. And price has nothing to do with a lens's UV-screening effectiveness.

Because it's a relatively easy process to coat *any* sunglasses (and even regular glasses) with the chemicals to filter out UV light, some optical specialty stores now offer this service. You can bring in your old pair of sunglasses to be treated rather than buying a new pair. The service usually costs between $10 and $30.

Besides screening out ultraviolet rays, your sunglasses should be chosen according to your individual needs. Gradient density lenses (which are dark at top and bottom, and lighter in the center) are good for skiing and boating, when sunlight can come from above or be reflected from the sun or water. Polarized lenses, which reduce the glaring reflections from flat surfaces, are good for driving, boating, or fishing. Ask an optician for advice. Let him know whether you'll be wearing the glasses primarily for driving, skiing, sightseeing, etc., and he'll be able to recommend the features that will be most useful to you.

Besides the sun, eyes are also vulnerable to chemicals such as chlorine and suntan lotion, which can cause chemical conjunctivitis or keratitis (inflammation of the cornea) if they get into the eye. You can protect yourself from these hazards by keeping suntan and sunscreen oils, lotions, or creams away from the skin of the eyelid and the skin directly around the eyes. Your sunglasses will also be good protection. If the chemicals do get into your eyes, irrigate them with an eyewash— many, such as Collyrium Eye Lotion, Laboptik Eye Wash or Murine Regular Formula, are available without a prescription—or simply use tap water. If the irritation persists, see a doctor.

To protect your eyes from water that may be contaminated and from pool disinfectants such as chlorine, wear protective goggles when swimming. Many of the new goggles and scuba masks now available are both comfortable and well-fitting, and it's possible to have them made with prescription lenses. People who wear contact lenses have the choice of wearing prescription goggles or simply wearing regular goggles with their lenses. An added benefit of wearing goggles: Swimming underwater with your eyes open increases the risk of viral eye infections, which are more common in summer or in warm climates; goggles protect your eyes against these infections as well as against chlorine irritation.

People with extended-wear contact lenses should take special precautions while swimming (hard and soft contact lens wearers should remove their lenses before swimming). To avoid losing your contacts or irritating your eyes, splash some pool water into your eyes before you start swimming. This will help the lenses adhere more closely. Some doctors recommend that the lenses be removed and cleaned after each swim to avoid bacterial contamination. Wait half an hour after you swim, or use saline drops, before you take your lenses out: They'll be easier to remove.

If the ocean, rather than a chlorinated pool, is your choice for swimming, take care to protect your eyes against gritty sand particles. If sand does get in your eyes, your tears will flush most of it out naturally. Splash your eyes with clean, cool water and blink several times to get rid of the rest. You may feel uncomfortable immediately afterward because of small scratches caused by the sand. A couple of aspirin and a cool washcloth on the face should ease the discomfort. But if you're still uncomfortable an hour or two later, you should see a doctor right away, because it is possible you have a deep scratch or a piece of sand embedded in your cornea. (People with extended-wear contact lenses should be especially cautious about dust and sand in the eye. Any time a foreign particle enters the eye, take your lenses out immediately to avoid corneal infections and ulcers.)

Finally, whether you wear eyeglasses or hard, soft, or extended-wear contact lenses, be sure to bring along an extra pair of lenses or glasses, and a copy of your prescription in case your glasses or lenses are lost or broken while you're away. Contact lens wearers must bring along all their "accessories," too, since it may be difficult to find the proper cleaning solution. Never use water that is unsafe for drinking to wash your lenses. If you use a sterilizer, don't forget an electrical adapter so that you can plug the device in anywhere. (You can also ask your eye doctor about switching to cold sterilization while you're away, since the heat sterilization machines don't always work as well when adapted to foreign voltage. But try the product out before you go away, since some people are allergic to the solution.)

It's no coincidence that people often refer to their voyages as "taking in the *sights*," and eyes that blur, tear, itch, or feel irritated can easily ruin a trip. But people with healthy, well-cared-for eyes, protected from the effects of sun, chlorine, and salt water, will return home with marvelous descriptions of the sights they've seen, and perfectly focused photographs to prove it!

6 | Making Peace with Your Environment

When you leave the confines of your comfortable office or cozy home, you come smack into contact with . . . the environment. And while it can be as friendly as a cool breeze on a summer day or a ray of sunlight through the trees, it can also be harsh and hostile. The same sun that warms your skin can make you ill. You may have journeyed to Nepal for the clear mountain air, but the high altitude may not agree with you. Every environment has its charms . . . and its hazards. But a healthy respect for and knowledge of the elements can keep you healthy while you enjoy them.

The Sun

The sun's danger to the skin and eyes has been discussed in chapter 5, but there are other precautions to take besides using chemical screens and tinted glasses to ensure sun safety.

Certain medications actually make you more sensitive to the sun, making sunburn, swelling, blisters, and skin rashes likely even with only brief exposure. Other phototoxic reactions (nonscientific types sometimes call this "sun allergy") include headaches, a burning sensation in the eyes, nausea, and vomiting. While you don't have to stay indoors to avoid the problem, you do have to use a strong sunscreen while you're outdoors.

Some of the drugs which can cause photosensitivity are, unfortunately, medications travelers are likely to be taking. Antihistamines (for colds, allergies, or motion sickness) as well as tetracycline antibiotics (such as Vibramycin, used to treat or prevent travelers' diarrhea) and chloroquine (Aralen, to prevent malaria) are among the drugs that may cause this reaction.

Other drugs that can cause unwanted side effects when combined with sun or heat:

- Acne medication such as isotretinoin (Accutane) and tretinoin (Retin-A)
- Antibacterials such as sulfamethoxazole (Gantanol, Bactrim, and Septra, the last two often used to prevent or treat travelers' diarrhea), and nalidixic acid (NegGram) for urinary tract infections
- Antidepressants such as amitriptyline (Elavil) and imipramine (Tofranil)
- Coal tar oils and shampoos used for psoriasis and eczema
- Some oral contraceptives (birth control pills) and other estrogens
- Topical corticosteroids, creams, and lotions used to treat many skin conditions such as poison ivy and other allergic skin reactions, insect bites, and itching
- Oral diabetes drugs such as Orinase and Tolinase
- Diuretics and antihypertensives (or combinations) used to treat high blood pressure, including Diuril, HydroDIURIL and Lasix
- Piroxicam (Feldene), a drug for arthritis
- Griseofulvin (Fulvicin, Grifulvin, Grisactin, Gris-PEG), tablets for ringworm and athlete's foot
- Tranquilizers such as chlorprothixene (Taractin), doxepin (Adapin, Sinequan), haloperidol (Haldol), loxapine (Loxitane), and the thiothixen phenothiazines such as Thorazine (chlorpromazine)

If you're in doubt about any medication you're taking, or just want to be sure before a trip to the tropics, a skiing jaunt, or any other outdoor vacation, call your physician or pharmacist for specific information on whatever medications you take. You can also go to the public library and look in a reference book such as the *PDR (Physician's Desk Reference)* to check the side effects of any drug.

Sometimes, a "sun allergy" can occur even when no medications are involved. Some fragrances contained in perfumes, colognes, aftershaves, and deodorant soaps, for example, can cause a skin rash in the sun. Also, certain foods contain substances that react with sunlight and cause a rash. These foods include lemons, limes, parsley, celery, and carrots; if you handle them before spending time in the sun, wash your hands thoroughly before you go outside. In many cases, the specific cause of a sun rash or reaction will never be pinpointed.

If you do have a bad reaction to the sun, the recommended cure is to stay out of the sun completely for several days, and, of course, to stop using the products that caused the reaction, if possible. But while it's easy enough to avoid your perfume on days when you'll be sunbathing, it's impossible to stop taking your diabetes medication for any reason, let alone a suntan. Wear a strong sunscreen or sunblock whenever you spend time in the sun if you must take a medication that causes photosensitivity. Also wear protective clothing, try to minimize exposure by staying in the shade as much as possible, and drink lots of fluids.

The sun has very visible effects on the body—suntans and sunburns—but it also affects the body in ways that can't be seen. Sunlight can alter the body's immune system, making you susceptible to certain viruses. One condition that can worsen with sun exposure is cold sores, caused by a herpes virus. Anyone who is prone to cold sores on their lips should use a lip balm with a very strong sunscreen and reapply it frequently to avoid recurrences.

With all these warnings, it would be easy to think of the sun as an enemy to be avoided at all times (as some dermatologists would have us believe), but in spite of some of its harmful effects, there are benefits to sun exposure, too.

Sunshine helps the body produce Vitamin D, which is essential for the absorption of calcium and other minerals. And since calcium intake and absorption may help prevent colon cancer and osteoporosis (bone thinning), sunshine is helpful in preventing these diseases, too. Certain skin conditions, including acne, psoriasis, and some fungal infections (including athlete's foot), seem to improve with sunlight. Some studies have even shown that sunshine is a natural mood-improver, because it suppresses the secretion of the hormone melatonin.

But don't take these benefits as carte blanche to bask unprotected. Fifteen minutes of summer sun every other day, and twenty to thirty minutes every other day in the winter, is all that's needed to benefit from the good effects and avoid the bad.

Heat

There are a host of medical problems containing the word "heat": prickly heat, heat cramps, heat exhaustion. All of them are caused, in one way or another, by the body's failure to maintain its normal temperature of 98.6°F. (37°C.) in the face of a high environmental temperature. Give your body some help in its struggle to stay cool and avoid heat illness.

As the temperature rises, so does the desire to start shedding clothes. But it's not just the amount of clothing that keeps you cool, but the kind, too. Loose is always better than tight (to allow air to circulate), and natural fibers such as cotton and linen are better than synthetics (because natural fibers "breathe"). Try to avoid tight collars, cuffs, and waistbands—anything that may chafe or bind. Stick to light colors, if possible, which reflect the sun's rays.

Perspiration is the body's main defense against the heat. The body can perspire more efficiently, and without depleting itself of essential fluids, if your fluid intake compensates for your loss through sweating, evaporation, exhalation, and urination. For most people, in the absence of strenuous exercise, the average fluid loss in hot weather is three pints (three pounds) daily. Drink lots of fluid—at least three pints (six eight-ounce glasses) daily—to offset what you have lost. Cold water is the best choice, because it leaves the stomach quickly and doesn't cause cramps. Carbonated beverages can cause gas pains, and alcohol and caffeinated drinks are poor choices in hot weather because, as natural diuretics, they actually increase fluid excretion. Don't rely just on thirst to regulate fluid intake, because it's possible to lose up to two quarts (four pounds) of water before you actually feel thirsty. Since your thirst is quenched before you have replaced the lost fluids, make sure you drink frequently in hot weather whether you feel thirsty or not. In fact, make it a habit to drink a glass of water before you go outside into the heat, another glass every hour while you're outside (and much more if you're exercising; see chapter 7), and a glass again after you come indoors.

In extremely hot environments, where it's difficult to drink enough fluids, or where water may not always be available, you might consider eating salty foods, such as pretzels or crackers, to help replace the salt lost from sweat. (If you are on a salt-restricted diet for high blood pressure or a heart condition, check with your physician to see if you can make an exception in very hot weather.) Most doctors no longer recommend salt tablets to their patients, since they can cause nausea and stomach upsets.

To minimize your discomfort, you might also consider altering your diet. If the fruits and vegetables at your destination are safe to eat, eat lots of them. These foods can help replace the sodium and potassium lost in perspiration. Try to avoid eating a high protein diet, since protein produces ammonia wastes that must be excreted through urination—causing you to lose fluid. If you are going to eat a heavy meat or protein meal, it's better to consume it in the evening, when it's cooler outside; that way you won't feel uncomfortable from the heat produced by digesting the food. Also, remember that many countries with warm climates, such as India and Mexico, have a national cuisine characterized by heavily spiced foods. These foods are good for you in the heat because they stimulate your body to perspire and cool off.

Because it's difficult for perspiration to evaporate and cool the body when it's also very humid outside, most heat illnesses occur when heat and humidity combine. Any kind of physical activity or exertion increases your susceptibility, as do some drugs and chronic illnesses. Heart problems, diabetes, obesity, and old age all affect the body's ability to dissipate heat effectively, as do some abnormalities of the skin and sweat glands. Alcohol, antihistamines, some tranquilizers, antidepressants, antinausea drugs, and amphetamines all hinder the body's ability to cool itself. Finally, lack of acclimatization—in other words, a sudden arrival in a very hot environment from a cool or cold one—also means the body won't be doing its best job of keeping you cool. If you're traveling from a cold climate to a hot one—for instance, going to Hawaii from Boston in February—it takes your body from two to six weeks to fully adjust. For most vacationers and business travelers, this means it won't be possible to become completely acclimated while you're away.

The following are the major heat-related conditions, their symptoms and treatment:

■ Prickly heat is an itchy, bumpy skin rash of pink pimples caused by blocked sweat ducts. The rash usually occurs under clothing, on the sides of the neck, on the upper chest, and in the groin area and armpits. Wearing loose, light clothing will help prevent this condition. The rash will usually clear in a few days to a week if heat is avoided. Or the rash can be treated with a calamine lotion, which will help dry it, or with topical chlorhexidine, an antiseptic skin cleanser (sold under the brand name Hibiclens). But no lotions or cleansers should be applied to the rash over perspiration, since the pores can become clogged and the problem become worse. People with prickly heat should drink lots of fluids and avoid strenuous exercise for two to three weeks.

■ Heat cramps are painful spasms that are due to a chemical imbalance; they are not common, but when they occur it is often in well-conditioned people who have had large amounts of water or other fluids to drink after strenuous exercise in hot weather. The cramps usually affect the legs, abdominal muscles, and arms; some people suffer from stomach cramps and vomiting as well. Heat cramps can be prevented by drinking adequate water *before,* as well as during and after exercise. Slightly increasing salt intake by having a salty snack such as pretzels or potato chips may also help. Anyone suffering from heat cramps should be moved to a cool place. Rest and fluid replacement are the best treatments. Add a teaspoon of salt to a large glass of water; drink half a glass every fifteen minutes for an hour. Stretching and massaging the affected muscles may also offer some relief.

■ Heat exhaustion (also known as heat prostration) has symptoms that mimic the flu: fatigue, slightly elevated temperature, headache, dizziness, giddiness, nausea. Patients are usually sweating profusely, and have pale, cold, and clammy skin. Sometimes, a person with heat exhaustion will also suffer from cramps, vomiting, or fainting. The fact that the victim is perspiring means that his body's temperature control system is still functioning.

If you feel any of the symptoms of heat exhaustion, get yourself out of the heat and cool yourself down: Remove tight or restrictive clothing, lie down and cover yourself with wet towels, sponge yourself with cold water, or take a shower if you feel up to it. Keep your legs elevated eight to twelve inches. Sip liquids. An ideal fluid replacement is a teaspoon of salt added to a large glass of water. Drink half a glass every fifteen minutes for an hour, sipping slowly. (If you vomit, don't drink any more fluid.) Do *not* drink alcohol or caffeinated drinks, which impair the body's ability to regulate heat. Heat exhaustion requires medical attention if the symptoms are prolonged, worsen despite treatment, or include vomiting, fainting, or convulsions. If you're in doubt as to whether someone is suffering from heat exhaustion or the more serious heatstroke (see below), treat that person as if he or she were suffering from heatstroke, and call for medical help immediately.

■ Heatstroke (also called sunstroke) is the most dangerous form of heat illness, and can be fatal. It may affect otherwise healthy individuals during heavy exercise in hot weather. Or it may affect the ill or elderly on a hot day, even without any kind of exercise. The body of a person suffering from heatstroke *usually* has stopped perspiring, indicating it has lost all ability to regulate its internal temperature.

When the temperature rises above 70°F. (21°C.) with high humidity (over 65 percent), or above 90°F. (32°C.) no matter what the humidity, young and healthy people should be wary of heavy exercise. And the elderly and chronically ill, as well as people on certain medications (many common cold and allergy medicines, antinausea medicines, tranquilizers and antidepressants) should try to stay in air-conditioned buildings and drink plenty of fluids.

People suffering from heatstroke usually collapse into unconsciousness. If conscious, they will generally be confused, disoriented, or in a stupor; they may also be depressed or suffering from a severe headache. They will have extremely high body temperatures—over 102°F. (38.8°C.). (The highest temperature reported in a survivor who suffered no neurological damage was 115°F.) Their skin is usually flushed, hot, and dry, their pulse racing.

Anyone suffering from heatstroke must receive medical attention *immediately*. Emergency care is directed toward helping the victim maintain breathing, cooling the body, replacing fluids, and preventing heart attacks and liver, kidney, and brain damage. Until medical help arrives, you can help someone suffering from heatstroke by bringing him indoors or at least into the shade. Undress him, and sponge his bare skin with cool water or rubbing alcohol, apply cold packs continuously, or place him in a tub of cold water. You can also spray a heatstroke victim with a hose, or place ice wrapped in towels over the groin and neck area. Use an air conditioner or fan if available. Continue this treatment until the victim's temperature is no higher than 102°F. (38.8°C.), and repeat the process if the temperature starts to go up again. But above all, make sure that medical help arrives as soon as possible.

(A trivia note: One of the most effective ways to cool a person suffering from heatstroke is to spray them with tepid water and direct a fan on them. Recently, a group of Islamic pilgrims en route to Mecca developed heatstroke. To cool them off quickly, they were sprayed with water, then fanned by a low-flying helicopter called in for the occasion.)

Cold

DRESSING FOR WARMTH

Dressing for the cold is like the dance of the seven veils—lightweight layers are the key to success. The air between clothing layers traps body heat, so a shirt and light sweater are better than one bulky sweater. Loose clothing made of natural fibers such as silk or wool, or the newer thermal synthetics such as polypropylene, are the most effective. Long underwear and a turtleneck under your clothes are especially good, because they fit snugly around the neck, wrists, and ankles, trapping warm air close to the body. Your outermost layer should be wind- and water-resistant.

Layers work for feet, too. Wear loose boots with several layers of socks underneath.

Keep body parts that are vulnerable to the cold, such as fingers and ears, covered. Even your nose should be covered in very cold weather. For hands, mittens are warmer than gloves, because they allow the heat to radiate between fingers. And although you've heard it before, it bears repeating: WEAR A HAT. About half of your body's heat can escape through an uncovered head.

Finally, keeping yourself dry is the best way to keep yourself warm. Being wet in cold weather is the quickest way to lose heat, and that's true whether you are wet from rain, snow, or perspiration. If you get soaked through after a ski fall, caught in a snowstorm, or feel a "cold sweat" next to your body, come inside as quickly as you can. Dry off, change your clothes, and you'll soon be ready to head back outside.

PREVENTING COLD EXTREMITIES

Fingers, toes, ears, and noses seem to feel the cold much sooner than the rest of the body. That's because the body tries to conserve heat in its core by reducing blood flow to the extremities and increasing blood flow to the vital organs, where heat is most essential.

Keep your extremities warm by keeping them well-covered. You can also rev up your circulation by moving, rather than standing still, in the cold. Jump up and down, swing your legs back and forth, and massage your thighs to get the blood flowing into the feet. Tuck your hands into your armpits to keep them warm, or do arm circles to get the blood moving.

To keep feet toasty warm:

■ Keep them dry. Use powder or a foot deodorant, and change socks often. When feet are cold and wet, the moisture drains heat from the feet, until both water and feet are the same temperature . . . and so the feet end up colder than they were to begin with.

■ Make sure air can circulate around your feet. Loose thick socks will keep an insulating layer of air near the feet. Shoes and boots should be loose, too, and should allow you to wiggle your toes with ease.

■ Try giving up coffee and cigarettes, or at least avoiding them before you go outside. Both caffeine and nicotine constrict blood vessels and slow circulation. The feet are the first to suffer from this diminished blood flow.

■ Once your feet are cold, you must warm them to body temperature as soon as possible. You should not rub your feet to warm them. Instead, soak them in lukewarm (not hot) water, starting with cool water and gradually running it warmer. Feet suffering from cold exposure will turn red as blood vessels relax and dilate; there may be some pain. But if you're suffering from frostbite (see below), which can cause tissue damage, the skin may remain pale, with a lasting numbness or pins-and-needles sensation. If color and feeling don't return to normal after about half an hour, see a doctor immediately.

Women seem to suffer more from cold extremities than men do, with some physical justification. Because women have more inner body fat than men, their insides are more insulated, so less heat escapes to their extremities. So while women may feel colder, their internal organs are actually warmer than a man's would be. And they're at a physical advantage, because they're less likely to freeze to death or suffer from hypothermia.

AVOIDING ALCOHOL

Just as alcohol is bad in hot weather because it causes fluid excretion and affects the body's cooling mechanisms, it is bad in cold weather for the same reasons—the body also uses fluid to produce heat, and alcohol interferes with the body's heating mechanism. Alcohol also speeds up heat loss by dilating some of the small blood vessels in the extremities. Your hands, feet, and nose may feel warmer, but they are releasing heat that your heart, brain, and other organs need more.

CHILBLAINS

Chilblains are itchy, red swellings on the skin that occur as a result of poor circulation in cold weather. Warm clothing is the best prevention.

For most people with chilblains, simply coming inside makes the problem disappear. Try to avoid scratching the affected area, since it can cause an infection. An ointment such as petroleum jelly may provide some relief from the burning and itching.

RAYNAUD'S PHENOMENON

Cold fingers and toes are an inevitable condition of winter, but some people—those with Raynaud's phenomenon—are extra-sensitive to cold weather. Raynaud's phenomenon is a circulatory disorder in which the small arteries supplying blood to the extremities (usually the fingers and toes, and occasionally the nose, ears, and chin) become sensitive to the cold and suddenly constrict, reducing the flow of blood. The hands or feet first turn white, then a dusky blue. As they recover they turn a bright red, and can feel tingly or painful. The condition most often occurs in young women.

Most people with Raynaud's learn to live with it and to take precautions such as avoiding cold, stress (which can also bring on symptoms), and smoking (which can further impair circulation). Because Raynaud's often occurs either as an early sign of or in conjunction with other illnesses, such as rheumatism and arthritis, patients with Raynaud's are advised to have frequent medical examinations. Severe cases may require drugs or surgery, although some doctors are now experimenting with biofeedback exercises to help Raynaud's sufferers.

Raynaud's attacks often last just a few minutes, although they can occasionally last for hours. To ease the discomfort of mild attacks, and prevent tissue damage during long ones, patients can rewarm the affected part gradually, either by simply coming inside and staying in a warm room, or by immersing the body part in water that is the same temperature as the skin, and then is gradually made warmer.

HEART ATTACKS

The cold weather makes angina (heart pain) and heart attacks more likely, especially when combined with physical exertion. Cold temperatures cause blood vessels to constrict, and since people with heart disease may already have blood vessels narrowed by cholesterol buildup, the heart may not receive enough oxygen. Also, the heart has to work harder in cold temperatures to increase circulation and deliver body heat. Anyone with coronary risk factors can take a few steps to minimize the dangers. First, always dress warmly when outside in the cold. Second, wrap a wool scarf around your face to cover your mouth and nose. The wool will warm the air you inhale, and your body won't get so much of a shock each time you breathe. Finally, avoid strenuous physical activity in cold weather.

FROSTBITE

Your extremities—fingers, toes, ears, nose—are the most vulnerable to frostbite, which is tissue damage caused by overexposure to the cold. Frostbitten fingers are actually frozen fingers. In the early stages of frostbite, the skin is red and painful, prickling, or itching. Signs of advanced frostbite include white, gray, or yellow-tinged skin that is numb, and feels hard and cold to the touch. The skin may also be blistered.

Frostbite requires medical attention, but in the meantime you can rewarm an afflicted area in a warm (104°F. or 40°C.)—not hot—bath. Remove any constricting clothing or jewelry, such as rings. Gradual thawing at room temperature is the next best choice. If outdoors, place a frostbitten hand under your clothes and next to your body, or wrap frostbitten feet with clothing or a scarf. Do not warm frostbite with a heating pad, hot water bottle, stove, radiator, fire, etc., as all can cause burns. *Do not* rub or massage a frostbitten part, or break any of the blisters, as you can cause permanent tissue damage.

Do not allow yourself or anyone with frostbite to walk on frostbitten feet, smoke, or drink anything alcoholic.

The frostbitten area will become pink as it warms, and the numbness will fade. Put sterile gauze or a clean cloth over any broken blisters, and between frostbitten fingers or toes. It's very important never to allow a frostbitten part which has thawed to refreeze. It's less harmful to leave an area frozen until medical help arrives, than to have it thaw and then freeze again, causing more tissue damage.

HYPOTHERMIA

Defined as low body temperature (anything below 95°F. or 35°C.), hypothermia sounds to most people like an exotic condition probably affecting travelers to Alaska and the Arctic. But it's important to realize that people are at greatest risk for hypothermia when temperatures are between 30° and 50°F. (− 1° to 10°C.). It's *wet* cold that is the biggest risk factor here. Left untreated, hypothermia can lead to organ failure and even death. When wind and cold combine—the wind-chill factor—hypothermia is also more likely. And hypothermia can occur after exposure of as little as half an hour.

Infants, the elderly, very thin individuals, and people with chronic heart, lung, or neurological problems, are especially susceptible to hypothermia. People who cannot move around to keep warm—such as paraplegics or people with severe arthritis—are also at risk, as are hypothyroid patients. Certain drugs, such as tranquilizers and barbiturates, make hypothermia more likely. Smoking, drug and alcohol abuse, or even recent alcohol consumption, also increase risk.

The symptoms of hypothermia include uncontrollable shivering, slurred speech, and mental confusion. The abdomen may be cold to the touch. Drowsiness and unconsciousness can follow. Skin may be pale, bluish, bright pink, or puffy. Temperature is usually too low to register on a regular thermometer. To help someone with hypothermia, get them inside and keep them dry by removing any wet clothing and wrapping them in a warm blanket. Socks, hat, and gloves are also helpful. Do *not* massage them or elevate their legs. Do *not* give them warm liquids to drink unless they are only mildly impaired. Try to keep the victim awake, and head for the nearest emergency room or call for help immediately.

High Altitude

Those voyaging to such cities as Mexico City, La Paz, and Cuzco (the takeoff point for Machu Picchu in Peru), as well as many skiers, may find themselves uncomfortable, or even seriously ill, with altitude sickness. The symptoms include headache, dizziness, shortness of breath, nausea, fatigue, weakness, and insomnia, and they may easily be mistaken for flu. In its most serious form, altitude sickness progresses to pulmonary edema—fluid in the lungs. Sufferers may act disoriented, cough and wheeze, even claim to hear a "bubbling" in the chest. People with cardiac or pulmonary problems are especially susceptible. But even young and healthy adult travelers are at risk. Approximately one quarter of all visitors to high altitude areas suffer some degree of altitude sickness.

Altitude sickness, also called acute mountain sickness (AMS) usually occurs within hours or days after reaching an altitude of 8,000 feet or higher, although sometimes as low as 5,000 feet. (When traveling in a country that uses the metric system, remember that 1 meter = 3.28 feet.) Low barometric pressure and the lack of oxygen at high altitudes are responsible because they lower the level of oxygen in the blood. As the oxygen level becomes lower, the body's cells swell from accumulated water, causing the symptoms described above.

A gradual ascent—no more than 2,000 feet a day at elevations of five to ten thousand feet, then no more than 1,000 feet per day at elevations of 10,000 to 15,000 feet—is the best prevention against altitude sickness, but in this age of jet travel, the slow route is usually not the one travelers choose. Even those who travel under their own power, such as skiers, hikers, and backpackers, may ascend more rapidly, especially if they are very fit. So everyone should take preventive measures against altitude sickness.

In Peru, when residents of Lima (which is at sea level) visit the city of Cuzco—11,000 feet above sea level, high in the Andes—they take special precautions. First of all, they often swallow aspirin before departure to help thin their blood. Secondly, when they arrive in Cuzco, they drink a local brew called "mate de coca," or coca tea. This tea is brewed with the leaf of the coca plant, the basis for cocaine. The tea is a mild stimulant (to combat fatigue) and also a mild painkiller (to fight the nausea and headache).

While Americans don't have access to coca tea, they can still use aspirin (check with your physician first) to help their bodies get accustomed to new heights. Further, some doctors prescribe a diuretic, specifically, acetazolamide (Diamox), to avoid fluid retention, make the blood more acidic, and increase breathing (the more air moving through the lungs, the less likely you are to develop AMS). Try to cut down on salt, too, to avoid fluid retention. And aim for a diet high in carbohydrates to ensure higher blood-oxygen levels. Finally, drink plenty of nonalcoholic fluids—1½ quarts a day—because the rapid, deep breathing that you must do at higher altitudes is dehydrating.

Make sure you are urinating regularly, and that your urine is clear (not cloudy)—both signs that your body is functioning properly at high altitudes.

Give yourself a few days at a high altitude to get acclimated. Eat lightly and try to avoid alcohol and smoking. Avoid strenuous exercise on the first day, then gradually increase your activity level. Skiers should be especially careful to take it easy the first few days.

But when symptoms of altitude sickness persist and worsen, the best treatment is a prompt descent of at least 2,000 or 3,000 feet. More serious cases may require oxygen. Ignored, altitude sickness can be serious, even fatal.

(Another trivia note: Mountain climbers have reported another effect of rapid mountain ascents, and they've dubbed it "Rocky Mountain Barking Spiders." The curious name actually describes a very mundane syndrome: flatulence. Apparently, the lower air pressure affects the gastrointestinal tract, causing gas bubbles. [For the same reason, flatulence can occur on an airplane.] But the condition, although possibly embarrassing, is nothing to worry about!)

7 | Sports Savvy

Beware the vacation athlete, who can overexert himself or herself even more than the weekend quarterback. Anyone planning a sports vacation should get into shape *before* departure, and use common sense to avoid the aches, sprains. strains, and breaks that can put a crimp in any trip. Going directly from sitting behind a desk all day to climbing the Alps can't be accomplished without pain unless you get yourself into the proper condition beforehand. And be sure to have a pre-trip checkup if you're planning a vacation with lots of activity. This is especially true if: a) you are older than 35; b) you suffer from a chronic medical condition that might interfere with the activity; c) you are generally inactive; d) you have a cardiac risk factor such as excess weight, smoking, high blood pressure, high cholesterol level, high stress levels, or a family history of heart disease or diabetes; e) the activity will be especially strenuous; or f) the weather will be exceptionally hot.

Preparing for the trip means trying to get into shape specifically for the vacation activity. For instance, if you're going on a hiking expedition, try at least to take long, brisk walks as often as possible for several weeks before you leave. If you'll be playing tennis every day on vacation, try to play a couple of times a week before you go. If it's impossible to engage in the same sport in advance—for instance, if you're going canoeing, mountain climbing, scuba diving, or horseback riding—get yourself into generally good shape by working out at a gym or health club ahead of time. At least if your body is accustomed to some exercise, a vacation schedule of daily sports won't throw muscles, joints, and ligaments (not to mention heart and lungs) into shock.

Another important thing to do to avoid injury is to make sure you have the proper equipment. Whether you are buying your own or renting, make sure that your equipment fits correctly and is well-constructed. And this advice holds true whether you're looking for a canoe, a bicycle, a tennis racquet, or just sneakers. If you aren't expert enough to trust your own judgment, find a store with knowledgeable salespeople. You must be able to have absolute confidence in your equipment before you allow yourself to brave the rapids or dangle from a mountain using it.

Once both your body and your equipment are ready, and you have arrived at your destination, use some self-control to pace yourself and your activities. Going gung ho from day one may mean that you have no energy left for the end of your stay. Worse yet, you could injure yourself. Even if you've been working out regularly before your trip, you should get into your vacation sport gradually. Keep telling yourself that you have a whole week—or two, or three, or more—to enjoy yourself, so there's no need to overdo it the first few days. Always warm up before any sport, and cool down before quitting. And always listen to what your body is telling you: If you feel tired, it is a message for you to rest; if you feel thirsty, stop and get a drink. Most important, if you feel pain, you must *stop*.

What you eat and drink, and when you eat and drink it, also affect sports performance and health:

- You should eat no sooner than three to four-and-a-half hours before strenuous sports and two to three hours before any exercise. The stomach needs time to empty so blood that should be going to the muscles doesn't get diverted to the digestive tract.
- Drink nothing but plain water within two hours before exercise or sports.
- Eat more complex carbohydrates than fats or proteins, which take longer to digest.
- Avoid gassy foods (like brussels sprouts, cabbage, cauliflower, onions, and beans) that can cause intestinal discomfort during exercise.
- Avoid alcohol and caffeine, which promote urination and can cause dehydration. Alcohol also affects the body's temperature-regulating mechanisms, and impairs coordination and judgment, crucial for any physical activity.

If you exercise alone (as many runners do), participate in risky sports, or have a medical condition, always carry identification with pertinent medical information on it.

When you're deciding how hard or how long to play, take your environment into account. The advice about dealing with the heat, the cold, and altitude, etc., from chapter 6 is even more important for athletes and sports enthusiasts.

Heat

In hot weather, try to exercise in the early morning, in the shade, after sunset, or in an air-conditioned gym. Wear loose, light-colored clothing that breathes (allows perspiration and evaporation), such as cotton or the new, mesh-fabric synthetics. Be careful about using heavy sunscreen products over much of your body during an intense workout, since they can make it difficult for the skin's normal cooling (perspiration) to take place. In high humidity, even low temperatures can cause heat disorders, because perspiration becomes less effective.

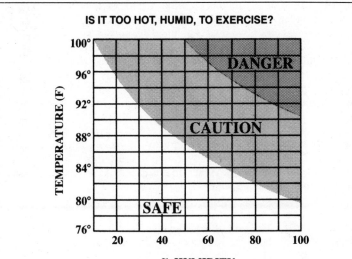

IS IT TOO HOT, HUMID, TO EXERCISE?

On a hot, humid day your skin cannot easily release all the heat your body produces during exercise, which can result in heat exhaustion (weakness produced by loss of fluids and salt) or heatstroke (a dangerous condition characterized by a very high body temperature).

Physicians at DUPAC (Duke University's Preventive Approach to Cardiology) recommend referring to this chart to determine when it's safe to exercise outdoors. When the combination of temperature and humidity are in the caution zone, you should watch for signs of overexertion and drink 16 oz. of water before you exercise and 8 oz. every 15 minutes during exercise. Do not exercise when the temperature-humidity readings are in the danger zone.

Drink water before, during, and after your workout. Drinking 8 to 20 ounces of liquid about half an hour before exercise will help keep your heart rate and body temperature down, and allow you to exercise more comfortably in the heat. Try to take a break every fifteen minutes to drink another half-glass of water; there is a 25 percent reduction in stamina with each quart and a half of water an adult loses.

Finally, weigh yourself after a workout and replace the weight you've lost, ounce for ounce, with fluids—two cups for every pound lost. At this point, fruit juice is quite acceptable, since it will also help replace lost minerals and carbohydrates. Replacing liquids according to how much weight you've lost is a much more accurate way to replace body fluids than simply relying on thirst. Up to two quarts of water can be lost before the body registers thirst, yet that same thirst will be quenched long before two quarts of liquid are consumed. A tall glass of water satisfies most people after a workout, but contains only about twelve ounces of liquid. The average runner can lose from one-half to two-thirds of a gallon of water per hour—that's four to over five pounds. Marathoners have been known to lose up to twelve pounds during a race, as have football players during intense competition or training. If fluid replacement is left entirely up to thirst, it can take several days after prolonged exercise to reestablish fluid balance.

Monitor your pulse rate when exercising in the heat. If you detect a sudden rise, it may indicate dehydration and a raised body temperature, which can lead to heat stress. In this case, take a break, sit where it's cool, and drink some water.

Never exercise in hot weather if you are ill, especially if you have a fever. And check with your physician to make sure that any medications you are taking won't affect your tolerance to high temperatures. Certain heart medications (diuretics, beta-blockers and vasodilators), antihistamines, and other drugs can increase the possibility of a heat injury.

Some experts say that it takes the body from two to six weeks to fully acclimate to hot weather from cold. And for those two to six weeks, strenuous activity should be avoided. Unfortunately, for most vacationers seeking sunny climes in winter, that would mean sitting out the entire trip. Common sense should be used in these cases to find a sports schedule that is comfortably paced and not overtaxing. You can help your body become acclimated to the heat by exercising for shorter intervals more frequently during the first few days. For example, instead of playing a full hour of tennis at noon, play for twenty minutes or half an hour in the morning and half an hour in the afternoon. Realistically, it's impossible to become an expert in any sport in the time that most vacations last. Better to be safe and healthy than try to be an instant jock and get hurt.

Cold

Cold weather causes muscles to contract, so there's a greater risk of pulling or tearing muscles and tendons when exercising in low temperatures. To prevent these injuries, a proper warm-up to stretch and lengthen muscles is essential, especially before sports like running or cross-country skiing. A cold weather warm-up should last from fifteen to twenty minutes, and should include jogging in place to generate body heat, as well as stretching exercises.

Dressing in layers is a smart cold weather sports strategy, since you can peel them off as your body heat increases during a workout. When you buy sneakers or other winter footgear, select them a half size larger than usual so you can layer socks underneath. And wear a hat to prevent heat loss from the scalp. On extremely cold days, you may want to put a light scarf over your mouth to prevent yourself from inhaling frigid air.

Although it may not seem so, replacing fluids is as important during cold weather as it is during warm, since the body still perspires during vigorous activity, regardless of the temperature. Consume beverages before, during, and after exercise, just as you would during hot weather. Water is still the best drink for this purpose. Do *not* eat snow to rehydrate, since the body loses heat when melting the snow internally. Eat frequent small meals or snacks to keep the body warm.

When you pull or strain a muscle from exercising in the cold, you must take longer to recuperate than you would in warm weather. Rest for at least a full week rather than just three or four days. Resuming exercise too quickly in cold weather can aggravate the injury or cause a recurrence.

The heart must work harder in the cold weather to increase circulation and deliver body heat, so heart attacks are more likely than during other times of the year. Middle-aged men, post-menopausal women, people with high blood pressure or high cholesterol levels, the overweight, smokers, those with a family history of heart disease, and people with any other known risk factor for heart disease should exercise with extreme caution in cold weather, and consult a physician before taking up a new sport or beginning a new program.

Altitude

Even world-class athletes have difficulty going from low to high altitudes. The rarefied, lower-oxygen atmosphere makes breathing labored when there's any exertion. People who attend aerobics classes regularly, for example, may be surprised to find themselves huffing and puffing just going up a small flight of stairs.

If you're traveling to somewhere eight thousand feet above sea level or higher (for example, Flagstaff, Arizona or La Paz, Bolivia), for a week or less, it might be wise to take a break from your jogging or exercise routine until you're on lower ground. If your trip is of longer duration, and you are loath to forgo your regular workout, you will have to wait a few days anyway, until your body has adjusted somewhat to the altitude (and the headaches, nausea, and insomnia that many people experience have passed). When you finally begin, start at a much lower level than usual. Instead of setting your pace by the *speed* to which you are accustomed, determine your workout intensity by the way your body feels: how out of breath you are, how fast your heart is beating, how much you are perspiring, and so forth. Even if you are running more slowly than usual, if your heart rate has risen to the optimum for aerobic exercise (the accepted formula is to calculate 220 minus your age, then determine 70 to 85 percent of that total), you will still be getting the same aerobic benefits. To take your heart rate, place your index and middle finger (*not* your thumb, which has a strong pulse of its own) either on the inside of your wrist or on the side of your neck, over the carotid artery. Count the beats for fifteen seconds, then multiply the number by four to get your pulse.

If you are going to be hiking at high altitudes, you need to take special precautions. A slow ascent from at or near sea level is crucial (if you'll be starting from a high altitude, you must give yourself plenty of time to get acclimated before you begin climbing higher). Experts recommend that hikers ascend no more than 2,000 feet per day at elevations of 5,000 to 10,000 feet, then no more than 1,000 feet per day at elevations of 10,000 to 15,000 feet. (Higher than 15,000 feet, the adjustment time varies with the individual.)

Anyone who experiences the symptoms of altitude sickness—cough, lack of appetite, nausea or vomiting, staggering gait, and severe headaches—must breathe deeply, rest, and eat quick-energy foods such as dried fruit or candy. Aspirin may help the headaches; antacid pills the nausea or lack of appetite. But if a rest stop doesn't ease symptoms, seek lower elevations immediately. Untreated, altitude sickness can eventually make its victim too weak to travel, and can be fatal.

All of the above advice is general, but there are specific health tips that apply to specific sports. No one should get involved in a new sport without good instruction and a pro's advice beforehand. And it's smart to read up on the finer points of any sport before jumping in. The following brief sport-by-sport guide will give you some ideas about what you should consider before embarking as a novice on a sports vacation.

Sports Guide

BICYCLING
In this sport, good equipment that has been properly adjusted to your body is the best assurance of comfort and safety. For long trips, special biking gloves are a good investment, since they protect the hands from blisters, and from some of the constant pressure on the ulnar nerve that can sometimes cause "handlebar palsy," a temporary loss of strength and sensitivity in the hands. (Bicycle gloves cost between $10 and $25 a pair.) Don't wear any item of clothing that could get caught in spokes (such as long scarves), and secure loose, ballooning sleeves or pants legs with rubber bands or specially made bicycle clips. Books, bags, and parcels should be carried either in a front basket, or secured to a carrier over the back wheel. If you must carry a shoulder bag or pocketbook, make sure it is secured to your body, and can't swing forward.

BOATING, CANOEING, SAILING
Besides learning the difference between stern and aft, it's important to remember that boating is as much a means of transportation as a sport. Just as in driving, therefore, absolute sobriety is crucially important for all crew members. Many, many boating accidents occur under the influence of alcohol, and drunk sailing is just as risky as drunk driving.

Also, don't assume that the cooling breeze and the salt spray eliminate heat hazards. Drink plenty of water to keep yourself hydrated, and use lots of sunscreens and moisturizers to protect your skin.

And of course, always be sure that your boat is properly equipped with life-saving devices.

GOLF

Golf is a pretty low risk sport, but common sense dictates that you watch out for swinging clubs and flying balls, and that you protect your eyes, skin, and scalp from the sun's rays. One hazard golfers face, albeit an unlikely one, is being struck by lightning. Golfers are generally out in the open, and the metal clubs they carry *can* act as lightning rods. Avoid playing golf when a lightning storm threatens, and if you are caught on the green in the midst of one, immediately seek indoor shelter or the inside of a closed car. If no shelter is available, drop your clubs and curl on the ground or squat with feet close together. Do *not* seek shelter under a tree.

HIKING

Hiking is a sport that requires very little equipment, but to prevent injuries during all but the most casual hiking on the smoothest trails, you shouldn't make do with plain sneakers or running shoes. Instead, purchase a pair of low-cut trail shoes, which weigh only slightly more than running shoes, but provide better support. If you don't want to make any investment because you are an infrequent hiker, wear a pair of sturdy leather Oxford-style shoes with a treaded rubber sole, instead of sneakers. For more demanding hiking—rough, steep, wet, or slippery trails—you'll need ankle-high hiking boots.

Hiking injuries often occur because of obstacles in the trail, such as roots, rocks, and logs. You should walk *around,* not on, these impediments to avoid injury. Take your time with hills, too, since these are another cause of hiking injuries.

People who usually wear bifocals should wear normal glasses when hiking, otherwise part of the terrain will always be out of focus, making injuries more likely.

If you haven't hiked before, or haven't hiked recently, take five-minute breaks every half hour to rest your feet, stretch, and drink some water. Never walk around barefoot in rural areas, however, since parasites can enter the body through the soles of the feet.

SCUBA DIVING

Most injuries in this sport occur not from equipment failure, but from panic among inexperienced divers. Proper instruction and supervision will prevent most injuries, as will making it routine practice never to dive alone. And of course, consult your physician about any medical problems before scuba diving. (Even dentures and false teeth can be a problem, making it difficult to hold the mouthpiece.)

One risk in scuba diving is developing a case of the bends: painful gas bubbles in the bloodstream that occur when a diver stays down too long or ascends too rapidly from depths of more than thirty feet. To avoid the bends:

- Never dive deeper than you've been trained to handle.
- Make your first dive of the day your deepest.
- Don't fly in an airplane, or travel by car, train, or bus through high mountains, for 48 hours after a dive, since the lower pressure of the plane cabin or high altitude, so soon after the increased pressure of a dive, can trigger a case of the bends.

Be alert for the following symptoms within twenty-four hours of diving: skin changes such as itching and mottling, joint pain, fatigue, headache, low back pain, abdominal pain, chest pain, dizziness, nausea, vomiting, shortness of breath, speech difficulties, urinary problems.

Such symptoms could mean that you'll need to repressurize and decompress in a hyperbaric chamber. Before diving anywhere, you should know the location of the nearest decompression chamber in case you require emergency treatment.

SKIING

An estimated half of all ski injuries are equipment-related, meaning failure of the bindings to release the boot after a fall or when a ski goes awry. So good equipment is especially important in this sport. Even if you're not an expert, you can test the binding releases yourself. Perform this check whether you own your own equipment or are renting skis:

To test the toe release, put your ski boot on and insert it into the binding. Bend your knee forward and inward. You should then be able to cause your toe to release if you continue to turn your knee inward. To test the heel release: Put on one ski and boot. With the ski flat on the floor, have someone stand on the tail of the ski. You should be able to step forward with the other leg (with no ski on) and pull the heel being tested upward enough with your own muscle strength to cause the heel to release. Repeat both tests on the other ski, being careful not to hurt yourself.

While even expert skiers fall, obviously beginners are much more likely to take a tumble. To minimize these occurrences, skiers should begin to get into shape for skiing six to eight weeks before the season. Exercises should be aimed at improving flexibility, endurance, strength, agility, and balance.

If you are a beginner, remember that skiing is *not* a sport to be self-taught; expert instruction is essential. The investment in ski lessons and proper equipment could save thousands in medical bills later on.

SNOWMOBILING

A good helmet and warm clothes are essential, but one additional risk of snowmobiling is damage to your ears. The driver of a snowmobile may be exposed to a noise level in excess of 90 decibels, which is enough to cause permanent hearing damage. Anyone riding a snowmobile should wear ear plugs for protection. (If you own a snowmobile, a muffler can help reduce the noise.)

SWIMMING

Drowning and paralysis due to diving accidents are the most serious risks in swimming, although both are easily preventable. *Never* swim if you've been drinking alcohol. Inexperienced swimmers should never enter water deeper than they can stand in, and *no one* should swim in an unsupervised area or brave strong ocean currents, especially alone.

To prevent diving injuries—currently the fourth leading cause of spinal cord injuries in the country—never dive into unfamiliar water. Don't even assume that the lakes and rivers in which you swam last season are the same depth they were previously; rainfall and other factors can change their depth from year to year. You can test the depth of water by jumping feet first into it from water's edge or a very low height. Then decide whether or not it is deep enough for diving headfirst. Risking injury to a foot or ankle is infinitely preferable to risking your neck. Never dive into cloudy or unclear water, since dangerous objects can be obscured. And be very careful when diving from boats or rafts, since anchors and cables underneath can cause injuries.

It isn't always necessary to wait two or three hours after eating before swimming again, regardless of what your mother told you. If you haven't eaten too heavily, if you're in good shape, and if you're not planning to swim very vigorously, you can jump right in. But if you're planning to swim serious laps, or you haven't been exercising for a while, you probably should wait. Swimming with gusto can divert blood and oxygen away from your stomach—where it's needed to digest food—to your muscles. And the result will be stomach cramps. (Note: Swimmers may not realize that they perspire when swimming, but they do, and they need to replenish fluids as much as other athletes and exercisers.)

Other risks of swimming, hard as they may be to believe, include polio, hepatitis, gastrointestinal illness, and parasitic infections such as schistosomiasis (so-called "swimmer's itch" is an early symptom of this condition). Swimming in water that is contaminated with organisms such as *E. coli,* enterococci, or microscopic worms—all found in sewage—can cause illness. Respiratory problems, skin diseases, or eye and ear infections can be the result of swimming in contaminated water. In general, ocean water is much less likely to be contaminated than lakes, ponds, rivers, and other fresh water. Chlorinated pools are usually safe. Be suspicious about swimming in fresh water in developing countries, especially in Africa, Asia, South America, and the Caribbean. On the beach in an underdeveloped country, always lie on a towel, mat, or blanket—never directly on sand or soil—to prevent parasitic organisms from entering through the skin.

If you do come in contact with fresh water that may be contaminated—whether you jump in on purpose to cool off, or get an accidental dunking—dry your skin by rubbing it vigorously with a towel, and repeat the action several times at ten-minute intervals. You can actually kill many microscopic worms this way before they penetrate your skin and cause infection.

In developing countries, the U.S. consulate may have a list of safe swimming areas. But even in the United States, there are streams and lakes contaminated with *Giardia,* an organism that causes diarrhea from one to three weeks after exposure. Unlike diarrhea caused by *E. coli,* giardiasis can sometimes persist for weeks or months if untreated.

Finally, some people are chronically troubled by outer ear infections, including "swimmer's ear" (otitis externa), a problem that can occur when the ear's canal lining is exposed to moisture and bacteria or fungus. The symptoms are a blocked and itchy sensation in the ear, a swollen ear canal, and, eventually, pain and tenderness when the ear is touched.

A full-blown case of swimmer's ear requires a doctor's care, but you can prevent the problem by drying out your ears with rubbing alcohol whenever you feel that they are moist or blocked after swimming, or even showering. Tilt your head with the affected ear facing upward, and squirt a dropperful of alcohol into it (if alcohol feels too harsh, you can mix it with an equal part of white vinegar). Wiggle the ear so the alcohol goes all the way in, then turn your head so it can run out. The alcohol will absorb the water, dry out the ear, and help kill any bacteria or fungi. As an alternative to alcohol, you can also purchase an over-the-counter product such as Ear Magic or Swim Ear, specially formulated for this problem.

People who often suffer from swimmer's ear, and will be spending a lot of time in the water, can prevent the condition by protecting the ears *before* they get wet. Put oily ear drops or lanolin in each ear before it is exposed to water. The drops will help protect the ears from infection.

Anyone with a perforated, ruptured, or punctured ear drum, who has already had an infection, or who has had ear surgery, should consult a physician before swimming, and before putting any drops in the ears.

TENNIS

In tennis and other racquet sports, besides stress injuries such as "tennis elbow," the big risk is being injured—especially in the eyes—by a fast-moving ball. In tennis, these injuries often occur to the person playing net. If you are hit in the eyes by a tennis ball, see an eye doctor *immediately* to make sure that you have not sustained a detached retina or other injury requiring treatment. To prevent eye injuries, invest in a pair of protective goggles. The best ones are made of polycarbonate plastic, which is virtually unbreakable.

Sports Injuries

Whether you've rushed into a sports trip unprepared, or you've followed all the advice carefully, accidents do happen. Minor problems such as aches, scrapes, sprains, and strains can be self-treated. More serious problems, such as torn ligaments, broken bones, and damaged joints, will require professional attention to prevent permanent impairment.

For the specifics on treating minor injuries yourself—and knowing when major ones require a doctor's care—see chapter 8 on First Aid. Of particular interest to the athletic vacationer: cramps, strains and sprains, shinsplints. Also, learn how to cope with heat and cold injuries, by referring to chapter 6.

Insurance

Finally, since sports vacations do carry more risk of injury than Caribbean beach jaunts, if you're planning a trip of this sort you should think seriously about obtaining travelers' medical insurance beforehand. When choosing a company, check the accident policy carefully to see if it specifically excludes coverage for injuries due to risky sports such as skiing, hang gliding, or scuba diving or other water sports; many do. Other companies will include sports accidents only for an extra charge, which may be as much as 50 percent more.

For more information about travelers' medical insurance, see chapter 1 for a list of companies that provide these policies.

8 | How to Help Yourself

In spite of the best precautions, accidents do happen. And since most accidents fall into the category of "annoying" and "uncomfortable," but not "life-threatening," they can often be managed by yourself. Why wait for a good samaritan (who may or may not speak your language) to come along, or waste time searching for a doctor for a minor problem, when you can learn to help yourself? Using the contents of the travelers' medical kit described in chapter 1, you can learn to treat such common problems as minor cuts and abrasions, bug bites, jellyfish stings, sprains, and strains. Learning how to handle the bugs, bruises, and sunburns of everyday life—and especially the traveling life—will also save you time and money.

Obviously, there are accidents and medical conditions that require emergency treatment or professional medical care. Head, neck, back, or chest injuries, shock, profuse bleeding, fractures, difficulty breathing, and severe burns require immediate attention by a medical professional. Unless you have had medical or first aid training, the best thing you can do for a victim is get help in a hurry. For advice on obtaining medical care when traveling, see chapter 12.

If you know that you'll be traveling in remote areas (such as the Himalayas) where medical care may not be available, or to underdeveloped countries in Africa or Asia where medical care may not be up to American standards, it is probably worth taking American Red Cross courses in first aid, including artificial respiration and CPR (cardiopulmonary resuscitation) before you go. The same holds true if you will be traveling with somebody whose health is impaired before the trip even begins (see chapter 11).

The travelers' first aid kit described in the first chapter of this book contains just about everything you will need to handle minor injuries. If you packed your kit correctly, it should also contain a small first aid manual. But just in case you've forgotten to include one, here's a miniguide to treating some common travel complaints.

The last section of this chapter includes tips on what action to take if you're caught in a hotel fire or earthquake.

Bites and Stings

INSECTS
Bites from mosquitoes, gnats, fleas, chiggers, and bedbugs are usually not serious. You can relieve the itching by washing the area with soap and water, then applying wet compresses, an ice cube, calamine lotion, household ammonia, or a paste made of baking soda and water or meat tenderizer and water to relieve inflammation and itching.

You should see a doctor if the bite becomes infected (which sometimes occurs from scratching). Signs include tenderness, throbbing, pus, redness and swelling around the bite, red streaks leading from the bite, swollen glands, and fever. Also see a physician if you contract a fever within ten days of an insect bite, since insects can transmit many diseases.

Tick bites require special care, beginning with the proper removal of the insect from the body. If the tick is not attached to the skin, simply remove it with your fingers and then crush it with a shoe. If, however, the tick does not come off easily, follow these steps:

1). Cover the insect with a few drops of mineral oil, olive oil, petroleum jelly, gasoline, or nail polish. The thick substance should suffocate and immobilize the tick within a couple of minutes.

2). Remove the tick with a pair of tweezers, being especially careful to remove the head and pincers. Crush the tick with a shoe or book.

3). Wash the bite area (plus your hands and the tweezers you used to remove the tick) thoroughly with soap and water, or alcohol.

4). Seek medical attention if the bite becomes infected. Also obtain medical care if a fever occurs within ten days of a tick bite, or if you develop a rash either around the bite or on the wrists and ankles (signs of Lyme disease or Rocky Mountain spotted fever).

Stings from bees, hornets, yellow jackets, and wasps are potentially dangerous because many people suffer life-threatening allergic reactions to them. And it's possible for someone to suffer an allergic reaction to a sting even if he has never reacted to one that way before, especially if he has suffered multiple stings.

To treat these stings: If there is a stinger remaining on the skin, remove it carefully with a tweezers, razor's edge, knife, or fingernail. Scrape rather than squeeze, since squeezing can cause the stinger to release more venom. Wash the sting with soap and water. Relieve pain with calamine lotion or a paste made of baking soda and water. Observe the victim carefully for signs of an allergic reaction, which usually occurs within the first thirty minutes and includes: skin rash such as hives, itching all over, pallor, weakness, wheezing, nausea, vomiting, and tightness in chest, nose, or throat.

If you know that the victim is allergic to bee stings, remove the stinger, then put a cold compress on the sting to alleviate pain and slow the absorption of the venom. Seek medical attention *immediately*. Individuals who know they are allergic to bee stings should carry injectable epinephrine. If the first signs of a reaction appear before you can reach proper medical care, the injection should prevent a severe, life-threatening allergic reaction until you can get help.

*   *   *

Certain spiders (black widows and brown recluses) and scorpions can inject their victims with powerful poisons that require immediate medical attention. In the meantime, have the victim lie still, with the bitten part immobile and lower than the heart. If the bite is on the arm or leg, tie a strip of cloth two to four inches above the bite. The bandage should be snug, but loose enough to permit blood circulation; a finger should be able to slip underneath the strip.

If the swelling travels up to the band, tie a second band two to four inches above the first, then remove the first one. Remove the band after half an hour, even if you have not yet reached medical care.

Apply ice wrapped in cloth (don't apply ice directly to the skin), or a cold compress to the bite.

ANIMALS

The first step in treating animal bites is to control serious bleeding, just as you would in a wound due to any cause (see instructions for Bleeding). Also, it's important that you capture the animal if it is wild. If you must kill it to capture it, try not to damage its head, since the brain should be tested for rabies. If the animal is domestic, take down the name and address of the owner. Once bleeding has been controlled, or if the bite is minor and there is no serious bleeding, wash the wound thoroughly with soap and water. Continue washing for at least five minutes; your aim is to remove saliva and other contamination.

Cover the wound with a thick sterile gauze or clean cloth pad. Press firmly against the wound with the pad, and place some ice against it. Try to keep the injury above the level of the heart while you are pressing. When even minor bleeding has stopped, cover the bite with a sterile bandage or clean cloth, and tie or tape it in place.

All animal bites require medical attention, because of the risk of rabies, tetanus, and infection. Let the doctor know the date of the victim's last tetanus shot. Don't use antiseptic or antibiotic ointments or sprays on the bite, or any medication or remedy, unless directed to do so by a doctor.

SNAKES

If you are certain that the snake is not poisonous, wash the wound well with soap and water and seek medical care. If, however, you are not sure whether or not the snake is poisonous, or if you know that it *is*, head for the nearest emergency room. Unless you can identify the type of snake responsible, try to have someone kill it so it can be identified at the hospital. Snakebites are rarely fatal, especially if medical attention is received within an hour. The pain and illness they cause, however, can be severe.

While on your way to medical attention, follow these steps: Have the victim lie still, with the bitten part immobile and lower than the heart. Tie a strip of cloth about two to four inches above the bite if it is on an arm or leg. The strip should be snug, but not so constricting that it cuts off the blood supply to the limb (there should still be a pulse on the limb, and a finger should be able to slip underneath the strip). Check the cloth periodically to make sure it remains snug but not too tight. Loosen it if necessary, but do not remove it. If the swelling travels to the band, tie another one two to four inches higher than the first, then remove the first band. Wash the bite well with soap and water.

Observe the victim for breathing difficulty and signs of shock; be prepared to give artificial respiration. Keep the victim calm, lying down, and covered with a blanket. If possible, someone should phone ahead to the hospital to alert the staff to the type of poisonous snake responsible for the bite.

CREATURES OF THE DEEP

Most jellyfish stings aren't dangerous, although they may be painful and swollen. If the ingredients are available, make a paste of meat tenderizer and water and spread it on the sting—the enzymes in the tenderizer will deactivate the poison in the sting. Calamine lotion or antihistamine cream will also relieve the symptoms; wash the area first with rubbing alcohol or diluted household ammonia. If the victim becomes short of breath or faints, get medical attention immediately.

One kind of jellyfish—the Portuguese Man-of-War—may cause a more serious reaction. Scrape off the tentacles with dry sand or a towel, and use meat tenderizer if it's available. Otherwise wash the area with either alcohol, vinegar, baking soda and water, or ammonia and saltwater. Do *not* use fresh water to wash the sting as it can set off any stingers that haven't yet fired. Get medical help immediately.

Remember never to touch jellyfish tentacles while you're treating yourself or someone else, because the sting of a dead jellyfish is still poisonous. Also, if someone is stung in the eye, do nothing in the way of first aid yourself, but see a doctor *immediately.*

If you step on sea urchins (ocean bottom creatures), you may wind up with a spine in your foot. You can treat the injury the way most doctors would . . . or you can try the method used by Caribbean island natives. Both are effective.

The straight medical treatment: Place a constricting band above the urchin spine and soak the area in hot water or use hot compresses for thirty minutes. Heat helps inactivate the venom. Remove the spine with tweezers, then wash the site thoroughly with soap and water.

The islanders' treatment: Pour lime juice or vinegar over the spine (it inactivates the poison by changing its pH). Then light a candle and drip hot wax over the area. When the wax cools and hardens, pull it off—the spine should come with it.

If symptoms are severe, if you don't remove all of the spine, or if the area begins to look infected, see a doctor for treatment.

If you are stung by coral or cut from stepping on barnacles or mussel shells, clean the wound out thoroughly with soap and water. Then see a physician about taking antibiotics, since these shells can be contaminated with harmful organisms that can cause illness or skin rashes.

You may be pinched on the hands or feet by a crab or lobster if you surprise one of these creatures while swimming. Treat a pinch wound by cleaning it out well, and seeing a doctor for antibiotics in case of infection.

The ominous-looking marine animals called stingrays or skates swim close to the ocean floor. They have poisonous barbs in their tails, which generally catch people right above the ankle or on the calf. Soak the wound in hot water, control the bleeding, and apply a dressing. Then seek medical assistance for a thorough cleansing and removal of any barb fragments.

Bleeding

MINOR CUTS AND SCRAPES

It's important to treat even minor cuts and scrapes when traveling, because they are a passageway into the bloodstream and body, and you must try to prevent infection-causing bacteria and parasites from entering. Treat minor cuts and abrasions (scrapes) by cleansing the wound and surrounding skin with soap and clean, warm water. Try to avoid using tap water in countries where the water is not safe for drinking; use purified or bottled water instead. If there is material embedded in a scrape that cannot be removed with soap and water, simply wash the area, apply a sterile dressing, and seek medical attention. Try to avoid touching a wound with dirty fingers, used handkerchiefs, or other soiled materials. You also shouldn't touch the wound with your mouth, or even breathe onto it since the mouth contains germs that can cause infection.

Hold a sterile gauze pad firmly over the wound until the bleeding stops. Then, depending on the size, cover with a Band-Aid or sterile gauze pad taped in place. It is not necessary to use an antiseptic cream or ointment, but one can be applied if desired.

According to the American Medical Association, a bleeding wound requires immediate medical attention if: it is *spurting* blood; slow bleeding continues for more than four to ten minutes; the injury is a deep puncture wound; the injury is very long or deep and may require stitches; a nerve or tendon is cut (especially if in the hand) and there is a loss of feeling or motion beyond the wound; the wound is on the face, or wherever a noticeable scar would be undesirable; the wound cannot be completely cleaned or contains a foreign body that will not wash out; the wound has been in contact with unclean soil or manure; the wound is from a bite (animal or human); there is a sign of infection (pain, reddened area around the wound, swelling). Also see a doctor if you have not received a tetanus booster within the last ten years.

In cases of large wounds, it is imperative that the bleeding be stopped as soon as possible, since blood loss can cause death in three to five minutes when large blood vessels are involved. Place a cloth pad over the wound and press firmly with both hands. If no cloth is available, close the wound with your hand or fingers and apply pressure. Use a bandage or cloth strip to hold the pad firmly in place. If possible, keep the wound higher than heart level. Have the victim lie down; keep him covered and warm, but keep the wound area visible so you can continue checking that bleeding is controlled. Do not give the victim fluids or alcoholic beverages. Obtain medical attention immediately.

NOSEBLEEDS

If the nosebleed follows a violent blow to the head, obtain medical care for the victim *immediately*. If it is just a garden-variety nosebleed caused by dryness, sneezing, or a slight bump or blow, have the person sit down and lean forward (to prevent blood from running down the throat), pinching his nose and breathing through his mouth.

While the nostrils are still being pinched, apply a cold compress to the nose and the surrounding area. If there is still bleeding after five minutes, the person can pack the bleeding nostril with gauze or clean cloth. The packing should be left at least partially hanging out of the nostril, so that it can be removed easily. Have the person pinch the packed nostril shut for another five minutes. If bleeding persists more than ten minutes, or if the person suffers from recurrent nosebleeds, consult a physician.

Bruises and Black Eyes

An ice bag or cold compress can relieve the pain and swelling of a bruise or black eye. If the bruise is still tender after twenty-four hours, warm, wet compresses can help speed healing. If the skin is broken, see the instructions for treating a cut or scratch.

See a physician for a bruise if: the bruise is still painful and swollen after a week; it involves a joint and limits motion; it worsens rather than heals. It's possible, for example, that a black eye is a sign of a fractured browbone. If a black eye impairs vision, or if the patient is particularly prone to bruising, also see a doctor.

Burns (Including Sunburn)

Most burns must be treated according to their degree: first, second, or third. This also applies to sunburns. Chemical burns, electrical burns, and burns affecting the eye require special care.

When treating any burn, never open blisters or remove dead skin. Never press on a burned area. Never put butter or household remedies on the burn, or even use ointments or sprays, unless under a doctor's instructions.

FIRST-DEGREE BURNS

These are red or discolored, mildly swollen, and painful; most sunburns fall into this category. To treat these burns, apply cold water to the burned area and, if necessary, follow with a dry dressing. Taking aspirin and drinking fluids will help relieve discomfort. A first-degree burn should heal completely in about a week. Medical attention is usually not required unless the burn is on the face, or if it covers a large area of the body.

SECOND-DEGREE BURNS

These burns are more painful and are characterized by a red or mottled appearance, blisters, and considerable swelling, which appears over a period of several days. To treat: 1) Immerse the burned part in cold tap water (not ice water) until the pain subsides. 2) Gently blot the burn dry with sterile or clean cloths that have been wrung out in ice water. 3) Apply dry, sterile gauze or a clean cloth as a protective bandage. 4) If the arms or legs are affected, keep them elevated.

If a second-degree burn is especially large or severe (for instance, if it involves more than ten percent of the body's surface, such as a leg or the back), it should receive immediate medical attention.

THIRD-DEGREE BURNS

These are the most severe; they appear white or charred, and often cause little or no pain. If there is a small area of third-degree burn in the midst of a larger area of first- or second-degree burn, treat the entire burn as a third-degree burn.

All third-degree burns require medical attention. Until it arrives: 1). Remove constrictive clothing or jewelry; 2). Apply cold, wet compresses with a clean (preferably sterile) cloth, and observe the victim for breathing problems. For small third-degree burns (smaller than two by two inches) you can put the burned part under running water or in a sink of cold water, but on larger burns, this treatment could induce shock. 3). Cover the burn with a sterile cloth or bandage. Do not give the person any fluids to drink.

ELECTRICAL BURNS

All burns of this kind should be considered third-degree burns. But before beginning any treatment, it's imperative that the victim be removed from the source of electricity. *Never* touch the victim until this has been accomplished. You may have to turn off a main power switch, or use a piece of rope or a stick to pull the victim to safety; but don't use your bare hands. And CPR may also be required for electrical shock victims. Seek medical help *immediately*.

CHEMICAL BURNS

These also require special treatment. For burns to the body, remove all clothing that has been contaminated by the chemical. Immediately flush the burned area with large quantities of cool water, and continue flushing for at least five minutes. Seek medical attention at once.

While waiting for medical care, you can relieve pain by covering the burn with cool, wet compresses.

For chemical burns to the eye, it's also important to flush the area with water. Turn the person's head to the side, with the uninjured eye higher (so that the chemical can't run into it). Hold the burned eye open with your fingers and flush it with large amounts of cool water from a faucet, drinking fountain, hose, or container. (If contaminated tap water is a problem and non-carbonated bottled water is available, bottled water is preferable. But *any* water is better than delaying treatment for chemical burns.) If water isn't available, you can use milk. Continue flushing for at least ten minutes. While waiting for medical help to arrive, cover *both* eyes (to reduce eye movement) with sterile or clean cloth pads, and bandage or tape them loosely in place.

Choking

Before you begin first aid for a choking victim, be certain that choking, and not a heart attack or other medical condition, is indeed the problem, and that the victim can't breathe. The easiest way to do this is to ascertain whether or not the victim can speak: A choking victim can't. A choking victim may also begin to turn blue, and will usually place his hand on his neck.

Once you've determined that the problem is choking, begin first aid—the Heimlich maneuver—immediately, since a person can die of strangulation in as little as four minutes. The following instructions for the Heimlich maneuver apply to adults, and to children over age twelve:

If the victim is standing or sitting, stand behind him and wrap your arms around his waist. Make a fist and place it slightly above the navel and below the rib cage against the patient's abdomen, with the thumb side of your fist down (against the victim's abdomen). Grasp your fist with your other hand and press it into the victim's abdomen with a quick upward thrust. Repeat several times if necessary.

If the victim is lying down, kneel astride his hips, facing him; for children age one to twelve, kneel next to the victim. Place the heel of one hand on the victim's abdomen slightly above the navel and below the rib cage. Place your other hand on top of the first. Press into the victim's abdomen with a quick upward thrust. Repeat several times if necessary.

If the choking victim is an infant less than one year old, the Heimlich maneuver should *not* be used. Instead, place the baby face down on your forearm with its head down, and the head and neck steady. Hold your arm down at about a sixty-degree angle, and brace your forearm against your body. Using the heel of your other hand, administer four rapid back blows high between the baby's shoulder blades.

If the back blows don't relieve the obstruction, turn the baby over and lay him down, face up, on a firm surface. Using just two fingers, deliver four rapid chest thrusts (similar to CPR) over the sternum.

If the baby still doesn't begin breathing, open its mouth and see if you can see the foreign body. Don't put your fingers deep into the throat unless you can actually see an object there and are trying to remove it. If the child still does not begin to breathe, try artificial respiration: four breaths by mouth-to-mouth or mouth to mouth-and-nose. Continue repeating all of these steps, beginning with the back blows, until medical help arrives.

Dental Emergencies

The advice below is intended to help keep you comfortable until you can see a dentist. If you are traveling in an underdeveloped country, or if you would simply feel more comfortable having your own dentist care for you, ask the foreign dentist if he can treat you for pain and swelling, and perhaps prescribe antibiotics to prevent or control infection. Then you can wait until you can see your own dentist after you return home (provided your return is in days, not weeks or months). It is an especially good idea to try and wait until you're home for treatment if you must have a tooth extracted. Not only is it painful to fly for several days following a tooth extraction (and other dental procedures, too), but the risk of infection is probably less at home.

BLEEDING IN MOUTH

Apply pressure with a clean cloth, piece of gauze, wad of cotton, or tissue to stop the bleeding. An ice cube wrapped in gauze can be held inside the mouth to minimize swelling. A wet tea bag applied to the bleeding area is also helpful, since the tannic acid in tea helps stop bleeding and promotes blood clotting. If the bleeding does not stop within a few minutes, get medical help.

BROKEN, CHIPPED, OR FRACTURED TOOTH

Swish warm water or salt water (one tablespoon salt to a glass of water) in your mouth around the tooth, then apply a cold compress to your face to minimize swelling. You can relieve the pain with aspirin, acetaminophen or ibuprofen. See a dentist immediately.

BROKEN DENTURES

Find and save as many pieces of your dentures as possible. If any of the appliance is wearable, wear it until it can be repaired. See a dentist as soon as possible.

DISLODGED OR KNOCKED-OUT TOOTH

Rinse the tooth gently in cool water; do not scrub. When you must handle the tooth, handle it by the top (the crown), not the root, so you don't damage any of the fibers that are necessary for reimplantation. Try to replace the tooth in the socket yourself (then hold it in place), but if you can't, place the tooth in a container of milk or cool water, or simply hold it in your mouth between the cheek and gum, being careful not to swallow it. Get to the dentist immediately. (If you don't have the tooth in place, you can apply a gauze compress to reduce the bleeding.)

If you can get to the dentist quickly enough, the tooth can usually be reimplanted: Up to a half an hour there is a 90 percent chance of success; after 1½ hours there is a 50 percent chance of success; teeth have even been successfully reimplanted after twenty-four hours or more.

LOST CROWN (CAP)

First of all, try to find your cap or crown. Many are gold-mounted and very expensive. If it's not broken, a dentist may be able to re-cement it in place. Rinse your mouth out with warm water or warm salt water. Visit a dentist for repair.

LOST FILLING

Rinse your mouth out with warm salt water. Floss between your teeth to remove loose particles. Applying a wad of cotton with oil of cloves—available in a pharmacy—may ease the pain. You can also take an over-the-counter pain reliever such as aspirin, acetaminophen, or ibuprofen. Visit a dentist to have the filling repaired.

TOOTHACHE

Rinse your mouth out vigorously with warm water or salt water. Floss between your teeth to remove loose particles. The traditional remedy for a toothache is oil of cloves (available in a pharmacy) applied on gauze or cotton to the sore tooth. Cold compresses on your face may also help the pain. You can also take a painkiller such as aspirin, acetaminophen, or ibuprofen. (If you take aspirin, be sure to swallow it whole, since if it crushes in your mouth it can burn gums and damage teeth.) See a dentist as soon as possible.

Fainting

Lay the person on his back and elevate his legs eight to twelve inches; you can put a pillow or cushion underneath the calves and ankles to achieve this. Loosen collars, neckties, or any other tight clothing around the neck and move hard objects away just in case the fainting precedes a seizure. If the person begins to vomit while lying down, turn him on his side (supporting the head with an arm or pillow) to keep the airway clear.

Wet a cloth with cool water and wipe the person's forehead and face (if cool water is not available, a cold soda can may be used). Don't *throw* water on a fainting victim, since he may breathe it into his lungs.

As the person comes to, keep him calm, and don't let him sit or stand up until he is fully recovered. When the person feels completely recovered, give him something to drink, preferably a beverage containing sugar, such as fruit juice or a soft drink.

If a fainting episode lasts more than a minute or two, keep the patient covered and warm, and seek medical advice.

Most fainting is the result of fright, hunger, or some other common reason. If you know the cause of a fainting episode, and it's happened before (for instance, some people faint each time they give blood), there's probably no need for concern. But frequent fainting episodes, or episodes that occur without apparent reason, warrant a visit to the doctor. Fainting can be a warning of a serious underlying condition, such as inner ear problems, diabetes, or impending stroke.

Foreign Bodies in Eye, Ear, or Nose

FOREIGN BODY IN EYE

Do not rub the eye. If you can see the object and it is beneath the lower eyelid, pull down on the lower eyelid and remove the particle with the edge of a sterile cloth bandage or clean handkerchief.

If the object is beneath the upper lid, grasp the eyelashes to elevate the upper lid and overlap the lower lid, permitting tears to wash the particle to the inner corner of the eye. Raise the eyelid, and with a moistened handkerchief or cloth corner, or cotton swab, remove the particle.

If you cannot see the object, try flushing the eye gently with lukewarm water either squeezed from an eyedropper or poured from a glass. (Or, if you happen to have it handy, you can use a commercially prepared eyewash.)

If you are unable to remove the particle, whether seen or unseen, or if the particle has penetrated the eye or is sharp or hot, cover *both* eyes (to reduce eye movement) with patches or gauze bandages secured with tape. Obviously, you will need to seek medical help *immediately*.

If pain and tearing persist for more than a few minutes after you have removed an object from the eye, also seek medical attention, since you may have a corneal abrasion.

FOREIGN BODY IN EAR

Have the victim tilt his head to one side and shake it gently to see if the object falls out. If not, seek medical attention; any probing done by a nonprofessional can damage the ear.

If an insect has entered the ear, a few drops of mineral oil (or olive oil, baby oil, cooking oil) will kill the insect, and a doctor will be able to remove it easily.

FOREIGN BODY IN NOSE

First, make sure the person is breathing calmly through his mouth. Have him blow his nose *gently* several times. If the object is small and smooth, such as a pea or a pearl (common in curious children), a sneeze may expel it (you can use pepper to set off sneezing). If gently blowing and sneezing don't work, seek medical advice. Do *not* try violent nose-blowing or probing the nostrils.

Poison Ivy, Oak, and Sumac

If you even think you have been exposed to one of these plants, don't wait for the telltale rash and symptoms to appear before taking action. Remove contaminated clothing carefully so it does not infect other areas; make sure no one touches the clothing (it should be washed thoroughly as soon as possible). Wash the exposed body parts immediately; rubbing alcohol works best, since it actually extracts the toxin from the skin. But even plain water, or soap and water, inactivate the toxin. Whether you use alcohol or water, don't just pat it on; *pour* it on.

An over-the-counter lotion with calamine or hydrocortisone should help minimize itching. Oral antihistamines may also help. Avoid scratching as it can lead to infection. Some people have especially severe allergic reactions to poisonous plants; be alert for signs of shock or breathing difficulty, and get medical help immediately if they occur.

See a doctor if: the rash is severe and includes blisters, or if it covers a large portion of the body; the rash is on the face or genitals; plant parts were chewed or swallowed. See a doctor, too, if the itching becomes unbearable. Prescription oral cortisone and cortisone creams can help provide relief.

Poisoning

Immediately telephone a local poison control center, emergency room, or physician for instructions. The type of poison determines the treatment. Have the poison container, with the label and any remaining contents, near the phone so you can describe them to the doctor. The doctor will need to know the victim's age, the name of the poison, how much was swallowed, whether or not the victim has already vomited, and how much time it will take to get the victim to an emergency room or medical facility.

If, however, you are in a foreign country where language is a barrier, or you are camping or hiking in the wilderness and cannot get to a telephone, you will have to take action yourself until you can get medical care.

For *most* poisons (see list below), the proper treatment, assuming the victim is conscious, is to dilute the poison by having the victim drink a glass of water or milk, then induce vomiting with syrup of ipecac. Syrup of ipecac should be given in the following doses: Adults and children over 10 years old—2 tablespoons (equals 6 teaspoons, or 30 milliliters, or 1 ounce); children 1 to 10 years old—1 tablespoon (equals 3 teaspoons, or 15 milliliters, or ½ ounce). Many experts advise that you not give ipecac syrup to a child under one year of age unless directed to do so by a doctor, but in an absolute emergency with no medical help available, give a child 9 months to a year old 2 teaspoons, or a child 6 to 8 months 1 teaspoon.

Afterward, have the victim drink one or two eight-ounce glasses of water, then lie down over the side of a bed so that his head is lower than his body to prevent choking while vomiting. If he doesn't vomit in fifteen minutes, give a second dose of ipecac syrup. (Don't give a third.) Save the vomited material for analysis.

If you don't have syrup of ipecac, you can tickle the back of the throat with your fingers, or you can place a spoon handle or finger at the back of the throat to induce vomiting.

The above treatment is advised for poisoning due to most medicines and drugs, poisonous plants, pesticides, rat or mouse poison, cosmetics or deodorant, perfume, and alcohol.

In general, you should *not* induce vomiting if the swallowed poison is an acid or alkali (household cleansers such as ammonia, bleach, dishwasher detergent, drain and toilet cleaner, metal cleaner, oven cleaner, lye, rust remover) or a petroleum-like product (floor polish and wax, furniture polish or wax, gasoline, kerosene, lighter fluid, liquid naphtha, paint thinner, turpentine, wood preservative). One way to identify that someone has swallowed one of these substances is by a gasoline-like odor on the breath, or telltale burns on the face, mouth, or throat. In these cases, you can dilute the poison by having the victim drink a glass of water or milk until you receive further instructions from a physician.

Also, don't induce vomiting if you don't know what was swallowed, or if the victim is unconscious, having convulsions, or has pain or burning in the throat or mouth. In any of these cases, you must follow medical advice given over the phone by a doctor or medical facility, or get the patient to an emergency room as quickly as possible.

Sports Injuries

Most sports injuries are treated by a series of actions known as R.I.C.E.: rest, ice, compression, and elevation. In other words, rest the injured part, use ice compresses followed by elastic bandages to minimize discomfort and swelling (remove the bandage if the pain increases or the skin turns pale, numb, or tingly). And keep the injured part elevated as much as possible while it's healing. An over-the-counter painkiller such as aspirin, acetaminophen, or ibuprofen can be taken if desired.

Obviously, some sports injuries are more severe, and require different treatment. A suspected fracture or dislocation, for example, requires *immediate* medical attention.

The following are some common, relatively minor sports injuries, and the specifics for their treatment:

MUSCLE CRAMPS

Stretch and massage the muscle. Apply heat (heating pad, warm bath, hot water bottle wrapped in a towel, or warm, wet compresses). If the cramp occurs after exercise on a hot day, see the instructions for heat cramps in chapter 6. If cramps can't be relieved, or if they occur repeatedly, see a doctor.

SPRAINS (PULL OR TEAR OF A LIGAMENT)

Sprains most commonly affect the knees, fingers, ankles, and feet. Use the R.I.C.E. treatment described above, and avoid weight-bearing on the affected part.

It's difficult to distinguish a sprain from a fracture; if you're in doubt about what you're suffering from, see a doctor. Also see a physician if: there is an almost total loss of function in the injured part, the injury causes the part to look deformed, pain and swelling persist longer than two days, there is significant swelling around a joint, or the patient is a child or adolescent.

STRAINS (PULL OR TEAR OF MUSCLES OR TENDONS)

Rest a strained ("pulled") muscle; do not try to "work the injury out" by exercising it, as this will probably make it worse. If the strain affects an arm or leg, elevate the limb to minimize swelling. Apply cold (a cold pack, cold wet compress, or ice wrapped in cloth) as soon as possible. Continue applying cold for up to twenty-four hours (with periodic removals, at least every twenty minutes, to avoid injury to the skin) until the pain and swelling subside. After twenty-four hours, apply *warm,* wet compresses.

See a doctor if the strain affects your back, if the pain and swelling last longer than a week, or if there is a near total loss of function in the injured region. Chronic muscle strain can produce tendinitis, which requires medical care.

SHINSPLINTS
Reduce your activity to a level that is comfortable. Take aspirin, acetaminophen or ibuprofen for pain if desired. Before any further activity, such as running or aerobic dancing, ice your legs with cold packs. If the pain is severe, if it lasts longer than a week, even with rest, or if there is any loss of motion in the feet, ankle, or lower leg, see a doctor.

Occasionally, travelers find themselves in a hazardous situation that is unfamiliar to them. Here are guidelines for minimizing the chance of injury to you and your family during an earthquake or hotel fire, two events that *could* occur during a voyage.

What to Do if You're Caught in a Hotel Fire or Earthquake

IN AN EARTHQUAKE

If you're indoors:
- Find cover and move away from windows, high furniture, and other dangers such as hanging plants, pictures, or mirrors.
- Move to an inside doorway, or under heavy furniture like a table or bed.
- If you're confined to a wheelchair, stay in the chair and move to an inside doorway, then lock the chair wheels and wait.
- Don't enter or exit a building.
- Be careful of falling objects.
- After the shaking has stopped, don't use an elevator, since the cable could be damaged. Be wary of gas or water pipes (since there could be leaks) and electrical wires and outlets (since there could be shorts).
- Wear protective shoes and clothing to protect against broken glass and other objects.

If you're driving:

- Stop the car as soon as it's safely possible. Avoid bringing the car to a halt under or near bridges, overpasses, utility wires, or other structures which could be damaged.
- Stay in the car until the shaking stops. The car will shake violently because of its suspension, but it is safe.
- When the earthquake is over, proceed cautiously. Avoid driving over or under bridges, overpasses, and other structures that may have been damaged by the quake, or could still be damaged by aftershocks.

If you are outdoors:

- Move to a clear area away from trees, signs, and buildings.

IN A HOTEL FIRE

- When you first notice smoke or fire, call the hotel operator *and* the fire department to report it. Give your room number to the operator, so rescuers will know to check your room.
- Stay low, since smoke and heat rise; the closer to the floor you are, the better you will be able to breathe.
- Grab your room key and go to your room door. Feel the door with the palm of your hand. If it is *not* hot, open it cautiously to check the hallway. If the hallway appears clear, head for the stairway (ideally, you should have noted the location of the exits when you checked into the hotel). Do *not* use the elevators.
- If the stairway is clear, not smoke-filled, begin descending.
- At any point, if you are stopped by smoke or fire, return to your room.
- If you have returned to your room, or are there because the door to the hallway was hot and you could not leave it in the first place, go into the bathroom and fill the tub with cold water.
- Turn off the heating or air-conditioning. Turn off vents.
- Soak towels in cold water and stuff them across the bottom crack of the room door, and over air vents.
- Open a window; do *not* break one, since you may need the windows later if there's smoke outside. If smoke enters the room through the windows, hang out a sheet as a signal and close the window.
- If your room begins to fill with smoke, go into the bathroom and close the door. Cover the crack in the bathroom door with a towel soaked in water. You can also hold a soaked towel over your nose and mouth to help avoid smoke damage to your lungs.

9 | The Female Traveler

Sexual equality or not, women have special needs when they travel—needs related to contraception, menstruation, and pregnancy, among other things. The rule of thumb in handling all these facts of life with a minimum of interruption in your schedule is the same as the Girl Scouts' motto: Be Prepared.

Menstruation

Women should consult their calendars carefully before a trip: If there's *any* chance at all of your period arriving while you are away, make sure you bring all the necessary accoutrements—tampons, pads, medication for cramps—along with you. This advice also holds true if your period is scheduled to come shortly after you're due home, but there's even a slight possibility that you will extend your trip. Bringing your own supplies is especially important if you are traveling to an underdeveloped country, or will be camping or hiking in the wilderness. And while you will certainly be able to find whatever you need in most developed countries and in tourist resorts, you're better off with a brand of tampon or medication with which you are comfortable. Besides, there's always the chance that you will get your period on an airplane, during an excursion into the countryside, or some other place where it's impossible to pop into the nearest drugstore. Carrying tampons, pads, or medication with you gives you one less "in case" to worry about, and eliminates the need for a possibly fruitless and probably embarrassing search.

But even if you're *not* expecting your period, it doesn't hurt to bring tampons or pads with you anyway. The stress and change in your schedule that traveling entails can temporarily alter even the most regular cycles. It's always best to be prepared, even if it means packing a few bulky boxes of supplies. This is *not* the area in which to skimp when you're deciding what to leave behind in an effort to pack lightly. Newer, compact maxi-pads, which are hardly bigger than the old "mini-pads," may help you save some luggage space.

One final note on menstruation: Many women are more susceptible to motion sickness during their periods. Even if your stomach usually doesn't give you any problem, take along an over-the-counter anti-motion sickness medication, or the prescription Transderm Scōp patch, just in case, if you'll be traveling (especially by boat) during your period.

Vaginal and Urinary Tract Infections

Many women suffer from occasional vaginal infections—bacterial vaginitis (also called nonspecific vaginitis), yeast infections (also called candida or monilia infections) and trichomoniasis. And while these conditions are usually not serious, the symptoms of itching, discharge, and burning can be so uncomfortable as to ruin a trip. If you've suffered from vaginal infections in the past, ask your doctor to prescribe medication you can take with you so if you have a recurrence, you won't need to suffer the indignity of an internal exam by a strange doctor in a strange country to obtain the medication you need. Different medications are used to treat vaginal infections, depending on the organism responsible for the condition. Yeast infections, for example, can be treated by one of a variety of antifungal agents, such as nystatin (Mycostatin, Nilstat), miconazole (Monistat), and clotrimazole (Gyne-Lotrimin, Mycelex-G). These drugs may come in the form of vaginal creams, tablets, or suppositories. Most of these medications travel well, and can be kept at room temperature. But occasionally a medication—such as Mycostatin Vaginal Tablets—requires refrigeration to maintain potency. In such a case, request a substitute medicine from your doctor, since it is difficult to know if you will be able to refrigerate your medicine while you are away from home.

Vaginal infections are more likely to occur in warm climates, since heat and moisture provide an ideal breeding ground for many fungal and bacterial organisms. You can reduce your chances of developing a vaginal infection by wearing light, loose clothing. Wearing cotton underpants rather than nylon may also help. Avoid tight jeans or shorts, wet bathing suits, and pantyhose, if possible. Douching, bath oils, bubble baths, and hygiene sprays can also irritate the genital area and make infection more likely. In the bathroom, wipe from front to back to avoid bringing bacteria from the bowel into the vagina.

If you are taking antibiotics to prevent (or treat) diarrhea, or for any other condition, you should know that these drugs can also make yeast infections more likely. Besides killing "bad" organisms, they also kill some of the body's normal, protective organisms, such as those that inhabit the vaginal tract and protect against infection. (Conversely, antibiotics—albeit different ones—may be used to treat vaginitis and trichomoniasis.) Women prone to yeast infections should consider asking their physician for an anti-yeast medication to use preventively if they are taking antibiotics.

Urinary tract infections (UTI), including cystitis (a bladder infection), are also common "women's problems." The symptoms include a frequent urge to urinate, a burning sensation upon urination, and, occasionally, blood in the urine. Be sure to take along the necessary medications—usually antibiotics or sulfa drugs—if you are prone to these infections.

Like travelers' diarrhea, the organism responsible for most cases of UTI is *E. coli.* And two of the medications used to prevent and treat travelers' diarrhea—Bactrim and Septra—can also be used to treat UTIs. Tell your physician if you are prone to UTIs *and* you'll be traveling to an area where turista is a risk; it may make sense to carry one of these drugs. (This advice is especially important to women on their honeymoons, or on any kind of romantic voyage with a lover. Sexual intercourse is one way in which these infections are acquired, and often women first suffer from UTIs when they first become sexually active. Doctors have even coined the term "honeymoon cystitis" to apply to these cases.)

Contraception

Contraception poses another problem for women when they're away from home. One of the first dilemmas for some women—those traveling alone or on business trips—is whether to bring birth control along with them. The answer is, unequivocally, "yes." If you're even debating whether to pack contraceptives—you should. Better to carry them home unused than to encounter a situation where you wished desperately that you'd had them with you.

Women with diaphragms or IUDs, or those who rely on spermicides, should not find that traveling changes their contraceptive practices. Women on the Pill, however, may have to make a few adjustments to compensate for time changes and travelers' ailments:

Make sure you have enough oral contraceptives to last the entire length of your trip and then some, in case your return home is delayed. Also, have your doctor write down the brand name and generic name of your contraceptive, so that you can give another doctor the information if you must replace the pills. Women on the Pill should always travel with a barrier method of contraception (spermicide, sponge, diaphragm) as a backup in case the pills run out or are lost, or in case you forget to take them for a day or two and have to use another method to be sure. (Ask your doctor what to do if you miss one or two days of the Pill. Some recommend that you throw away the pills you forgot to take, and then continue the cycle as usual. Others recommend that if you skip one day, you take two pills the next day, if you skip two days, take two pills for the next two days . . . and then continue the cycle as usual. But in any of these cases, you must use a backup method of contraception for the rest of that menstrual cycle. If you miss more than two days of the Pill, don't take any more medication from that pack. Use some other form of contraception for the rest of the cycle. Then start a new pill cycle.)

Illness and certain medications can also make the Pill less effective, and can make it necessary to use a backup method of contraception. For instance, vomiting and diarrhea (the traveler's curse) can reduce the Pill's absorption in the body, and render it ineffective. If you are sick for more than a day, use a backup method to be safe. Antibiotics can also occasionally interfere with the Pill's effectiveness. If you are taking antibiotics to prevent or treat travelers' diarrhea, or for any other reason, check with your doctor before your trip to see if your oral contraceptive will be affected. In general, the new low-dose pills are most susceptible to the effects of antibiotics.

Dealing with time changes can be confusing for many women on the Pill. Depending on the length of the time difference and the type of oral contraceptive you take, you may simply be able to continue your usual habits. For instance, women taking combination pills should be able to continue taking them at bedtime, no matter where they are or how great the time difference. But certain oral contraceptives, such as progestin-only Pills (mini-pills), must be taken every twenty-four hours to be effective. If you usually take the Pill at bedtime, you may wind up having to take it in the middle of the night or very early in the morning, depending on the time change. If you are traveling for a considerable length of time, switch the timing gradually—no more than an hour per dose, so that you are taking the Pill every twenty-three hours instead of every twenty-four—until you are once again taking the Pill when it is convenient for you. You'll need to switch back just as gradually when you return home. (For short trips—less than a week—it makes more sense to keep yourself on home time, at least as far as taking the Pill goes.) For safety, check with your physician for the specifics about your prescription and the time difference you'll be experiencing.

No matter what type of contraception you use, if you lose or run out of it, you will have to find a replacement. In most countries, over-the-counter barrier methods, such as condoms and spermicidal creams, are readily available. (The few countries that are exceptions, such as fundamentalist Islamic nations, are not generally popular tourist or even business destinations.) In fact, most Americans will find it easier to buy birth control over-the-counter abroad than at home. In Scandinavia, for example, condoms are sold in vending machines. And in many developing countries, it's even possible to purchase oral contraceptives without a prescription (though it's not wise to buy or take these without a doctor's recommendation).

If you'll be away for longer than a couple of weeks, you should probably take a few extra precautions to ensure that you don't find yourself without an acceptable method of contraception. Call the International Planned Parenthood Federation (IPPF) in New York City at (212) 679-2230 before your trip to find out the address and phone number of the nearest family planning office at your destination. The information is included in IPPF's booklet "World List of Family Planning Addresses." If you need to consult one of these addresses while you're away—for instance, if you run out of contraceptives or simply need family planning advice—they should be able to help. IPPF also publishes a "Directory of Contraceptives," a copy of which should be in most international family planning offices. (Local Planned Parenthood offices may not have this information.) This booklet lists the contraceptive brand names (and their chemical formulations) available in most countries of the world. The list will help a foreign doctor to provide you with a replacement contraceptive identical or similar to the one you have finished or lost.

Pregnancy

As modern medicine continues to revise its view of pregnancy from a "disease" that requires treatment, to the special—but healthy—condition that it is, the recommended constraints on a pregnant woman's activities become fewer and fewer. Nevertheless, traveling during pregnancy still requires precautions.

The first consideration is timing. Most specialists recommend that pregnant women travel during their second trimester—the fourth through sixth months of pregnancy. It is during these three months that most pregnant women feel most comfortable, since the nausea and morning sickness of the first trimester have ended, but the heaviness, bulkiness, and fatigue of the last trimester have not yet arrived. Also, the middle three months are medically the safest time for travel, because miscarriages and complications are least likely to occur (spontaneous abortions usually occur early in pregnancy, while premature labor or ruptured membranes are almost always after the sixth month). Since the biggest risk in traveling during pregnancy is of developing a complication and not being able to find adequate medical care, it makes sense to plan travel for the middle trimester. Finally, nearly all obstetricians recommend that any woman with a high-risk pregnancy, or anyone experiencing complications, avoid air travel throughout the entire nine months, and that *all* pregnant women avoid air travel after the eighth month, to avoid giving birth 35,000 feet over the Atlantic with the nearest doctor thousands of miles away. (Some airlines refuse to accept a woman who is more than 32 weeks pregnant as a passenger without a doctor's certificate.)

Given these restrictions, it's still possible to plan a trip around a pregnancy. Since the timing is fixed, the next decision is the place. The distance of your destination isn't as important as its health conditions. Pregnant women should try to avoid any country experiencing an epidemic or outbreak of a contagious disease (such as measles), as well as any country requiring vaccinations or other precautions that could be harmful to the developing fetus.

The effects of many vaccines—especially live vaccines—on the developing fetus are not yet known; they should be avoided if possible during pregnancy. Measles, mumps, and rubella vaccines should *not* be given to pregnant women. Pregnant women should also try to avoid many of the vaccines often recommended for travelers, although if the risk of disease exposure is high, and the risk to the fetus from the disease outweighs the risk from the vaccine, they can be given. For instance, if a woman must travel (because of business or family obligation) to a place experiencing an epidemic or outbreak of yellow fever, she can receive the vaccine. Other vaccines that fall into this category (that is, can be given during pregnancy, but only if absolutely necessary) include: polio, cholera, typhoid, rabies, plague, and meningococcal meningitis. Even so, these vaccines should not be administered until the second or third trimester, and a vaccine made of killed bacteria or inactivated viruses (which can no longer cause disease) is preferable to a live vaccine. Finally, hepatitis B vaccine, tetanus-diphtheria vaccine, and flu and pneumonia vaccines are considered safe during pregnancy, as is administration of immune globulins (if exposure to measles, hepatitis A or B, rabies, or tetanus is likely). Again, it's always best to wait until the second or third trimester before receiving these vaccines.

Pregnant women must also be cautious about drugs used to help prevent malaria, and if possible pregnant women should avoid travel to areas where malaria is endemic. Malaria prophylaxis with Fansidar (a drug sometimes used to prevent disease from strains of malaria resistant to chloroquine, the medication usually recommended) can be hazardous during pregnancy. Chloroquine (Aralen) is considered safe for pregnant women to take, but again, is only recommended when the risk of contracting the disease is high.

Pregnant women should not take antibiotics to prevent travelers' diarrhea.

To be absolutely safe, many obstetricians advise that pregnant women avoid traveling to *any* underdeveloped country, both to avoid exposure to disease, and to avoid being caught in a situation where urgent medical care is required but unavailable.

Once time and place are decided, the next choice is the means of transportation. Airplane travel is recommended because it is quickest, but pregnant women should be certain to travel in a plane that is pressurized (and indeed, just about all commercial planes are). An aisle or bulkhead seat will be most comfortable, because they allow easy access to the lavatories without the need to climb over other passengers. Fasten the seatbelt snugly across your upper thighs and under your tummy, so that there is no pressure on the womb. Getting up every forty-five minutes or so to move and walk around will help your circulation.

If you are making a shorter trip, choose a train over a bus, since the aisles will allow you greater movement. If you go by car, stop frequently—at least every two hours—so that you can walk around. When using a car's shoulder harness/seatbelt combination, make sure the lap belt fits snugly across your upper thighs or pelvic bones and under your tummy, and that the shoulder strap is between your breasts. Since pregnant women are more susceptible to motion sickness and nausea, it may be wise to avoid boats as a means of transportation. If you can, postpone a vacation cruise until after the baby is born. To avoid motion sickness during any voyage, eat lightly and carry a supply of bland crackers (you should not take anti-motion sickness medication to combat nausea unless you check with your physician first).

When you pack for your trip, include loose, comfortable clothing, and, especially, comfortable shoes. Bring along a strong sunscreen, since your skin may be more sensitive to the sun during pregnancy. Make sure your itinerary is not too taxing—it's important to sleep, relax, and avoid undue stress. Also, be careful of your diet. The tendency on vacation is to eat unfamiliar foods or to overeat. Remember that your diet is more important than ever now, and not even tempting foreign foods or resort buffets should sway you from your healthy habits during pregnancy. Make sure you drink plenty of fluids.

Finally, and most important: Make your obstetrician aware of your travel plans and itinerary, and follow his or her advice. Don't have *any* vaccinations or take *any* medication without your doctor's "okay." This is true for lactating (breast-feeding) women, also. You should also see if your obstetrician can give you the name of a good doctor or hospital at your destination in case of emergency. If not, it would be smart to sign up with IAMAT or Intermedic (for a list of English-speaking doctors around the world), or one of the travelers' insurance plans described in chapter 1.

10 | The Littlest Travelers

Children are not just "little adults," and making sure they, too, stay healthy while traveling involves more than simply scaling down the advice for grown-ups. Most of the information in this book *can* be adapted for children, however.

For instance, parents packing the *travelers' medical kit* (described in chapter 1) for themselves, can simply make a couple of additions to ensure that their children will also have the necessary supplies:

- Include a painkiller especially for children, such as Children's Tylenol (acetaminophen). (Be careful about giving children aspirin, because of the increased risk of Reye's syndrome.)
- Add whatever medicine you regularly give your children for colds and coughs, such as Bayer Children's Cold Tablets, Benadryl, Benylin, Children's CoTylenol, Contact Jr. Children's Cold Medicine, Dimetane, Dimetapp, Pediacare, Robitussin, Romilar Children's Cough Syrup or Sudafed.
- Add extra Band-Aids℗ to cope with youngsters' many cuts and scrapes.
- If you have young children, add a 1 ounce bottle of syrup of ipecac in case of accidental poisoning. (See chapter 8 on First Aid for instructions on using syrup of ipecac.)
- Take along Pedialyte, to replace the water and minerals lost from diarrhea or vomiting, if you'll be traveling to an area where turista may be a problem. (Pedialyte, available without a prescription, comes in 8-ounce glass bottles and quart plastic bottles. Once opened it must be refrigerated immediately and used within 48 hours.)

- For long car or boat trips, take along a motion sickness medication that children can use. Dramamine makes a cherry-flavored liquid that is especially good for kids.
- If your child is prone to ear infections or any other medical problem, take along the medication your pediatrician usually prescribes. You may have to call your doctor for a prescription before you leave.
- Finally, if your child takes prescription medicines, make sure you have more than enough to last the duration of your trip, since it may be difficult to obtain the same medication abroad.

Vaccination and Immunization

Before any trip, children's routine immunizations should be up to date. These include diphtheria, whooping cough (pertussis), tetanus, polio, measles, mumps, German measles, plus the new *Haemophilus influenzae* type B vaccine. Then, depending on where you are going, your children—like yourself—may need supplemental vaccines. When yellow fever or cholera vaccines are required for entrance into a certain country, they are required for children over one year of age, too. The yellow fever vaccine can be given to children aged six months and up, and is recommended if traveling to an infected area. Children can sometimes be exempt from receiving the cholera vaccine, however, since it is not considered very effective. A note from your physician may be all that is needed to waive this requirement.

When traveling to an area where rabies is present, ask your pediatrician about having your children vaccinated, since their natural curiosity puts them at greater risk than adults. Rabies-*free* areas include: Bermuda and many of the Caribbean islands, Iceland, Ireland, Malta, Norway, Spain, Sweden, Suriname, Uruguay, the United Kingdom, Australia, New Zealand, Japan, Taiwan, and many of the South Pacific islands. It's important to know, however, that even someone who has received the rabies vaccine requires additional medical treatment if exposed to the disease.

Children older than one year can receive the typhoid vaccine if necessary. And children who will be traveling to an area with malaria should take prophylactic medication (although in a much smaller dose than an adult's). Depending on your child's age, the recommended dose of chloroquine (Aralen) to prevent malaria is given in fractions (such as one-eighth) of a pill. You may need your pharmacist's help dividing the pills to ensure an accurate and correct dosage.

I.D.'s for Curious Kids

Children are ideal travelers: inquisitive, open-minded . . . and filled with wanderlust. That sense of adventure often leads them to stray in a crowded airline terminal or amusement park, much to their parents' horror. A child who knows his name, address, and phone number can quickly be reunited with his parents . . . if he's close to home. But when a family travels abroad, even an older child may not be able to communicate with airline officials, policemen, information officers, or anyone else who can help him. To bridge the language barrier, have your young children wear or carry some form of identification while traveling. Besides the child's (and your) name and address, the identification should include your travel itinerary, complete with plane schedules and hotel names. You will want to provide all the information authorities will need either to page you, or to locate you physically, if they find your child. Some parents also include a small photo of themselves, so the authorities can identify them accurately when they come to collect their child.

To make it easy for a youngster to carry this identification, you can write or type the information on a small card, and have it laminated so it can fit in a pocket without getting bent. Or you can write the information on a piece of paper and slip it in a pretty purse or locket for your daughter; a large, plastic toy locket should be big enough to include a sheet of paper. Easiest of all, you can follow the time-honored tradition of simply taping a piece of paper to your child's shirt (although only very young children will tolerate this without embarrassment).

You can also purchase an identification tag that is especially well suited for children. The Alert-Along Medical I.D. Tag is a plastic identification tag that can be worn around the neck, or even tucked into the laces of a child's shoes or sneakers. You can send away for the tag by writing to: Alert-Along Medical I.D. Tag, The Weiss Works, P.O. Box 374, Elkhart, IN 46515. Or call: (219) 294-2790. The tags cost $2 for one, or $5 for three.

Tips for Handling Common Travelers' Complaints

JET LAG

Children, with their endless stores of energy, do not seem to suffer from jet lag as much as do their poor parents, who not only have to cope with jet lag themselves, but must try to keep up with their active children. So it's not necessary for a child to try most of the anti-jet lag measures mentioned in chapter 2, such as the anti-jet lag diet or the light-exposure modification schedule. Still, it's not a bad idea to help children adjust to a time difference by changing their sleeping hours gradually before a trip, so that by the time the family arrives at its destination, everyone has a headstart at adapting to local time. For instance, if you will be traveling from New York to London—where the time is five hours ahead—have your child go to sleep an hour earlier than usual, and wake up an hour earlier, for a few days before the trip. (Since you can do the same thing to help yourself adjust, it shouldn't be a problem to have a child waking up at five o'clock in the morning.) Try to get the entire family onto local time as soon as you arrive. While it's better not to take naps, if your children are exhausted, you won't have any choice but to let them sleep. But in general, the excitement of traveling will keep youngsters wide awake.

MOTION SICKNESS

Children under two are the least likely of all people to suffer from motion sickness . . . but children between the ages of two and twelve are the most likely. You can help youngsters this age avoid discomfort, no matter what the means of transportation. In a car, have children sit on a pillow or, if they're small enough, in a car seat that boosts them high. They should be able to see where they're going. Like adults, if children can anticipate the vehicle's movement, their inner ears will compensate and they will be less likely to get queasy. Keeping car windows slightly open so that there is a constant supply of fresh air also helps.

If you'll be taking a boat trip, consider giving your child an anti-motion sickness medication. Cherry-flavored Dramamine Liquid is especially good, and can be given to children aged two and over. Otherwise, follow the directions for children's dosages on other motion sickness medication packages. All packages of Dramamine, cherry-flavored and regular, carry directions for children's doses, as do Benadryl and Marezine. Some anti-motion sickness medications, how-ever, such as Bonine and Antivert (which contain the antihistamine meclizine) should be used with caution, or not at all, in children under twelve. Unless a package specifically lists children's dosages, or you ask your child's doctor, children under twelve should not take an adult motion sickness medication.

AIRPLANE EARACHES

Anyone who's ever been on a plane with infants on board knows how they react to takeoff and landing: they usually cry. And the reason they're unhappy is that their ears hurt from the change in pressure. Babies have narrower eustachian tubes than adults, and their nasal passages are frequently clogged; hence they often suffer even more from air travel. And worse than the discomfort, the change in air pressure can cause a eustachian tube blockage, which can turn into a full-blown ear infection about three days later. Then parents will have a sick, miserable child on their hands right in the middle of their vacation.

Adults ease eardrum pressure by chewing gum, sucking hard candies, or yawning. Babies can achieve the same effect by nursing or sucking a bottle or pacifier during takeoff and landing. Carry bottles filled with your baby's favorite liquid on board, so that he or she is not reluctant to drink. The constant swallowing helps equalize the pressure on both sides of the eardrums, relieving the pain.

Alternatively, you can ask your pediatrician about giving your baby a combination antihistamine and decongestant about an hour before the flight, and then again an hour before landing (if the first dose has worn off). The decongestant will help keep the eustachian tubes clear, and the antihistamine will make the baby slightly drowsy, so he is less likely to be restless or to cry.

Older children can follow the same methods adults do to avoid discomfort: chewing gum, sucking candy, yawning, or doing the modified Valsalva's maneuver (pinching the nostrils together and then trying to blow gently out of them, unblocking the ears). Alternately, they, too, can take an over-the-counter decongestant, such as Children's Sudafed Liquid.

SEATBELT SAFETY

No matter how you're traveling, never buckle an infant into a seatbelt with an adult. Whether your plane hits some air turbulence, or the car in which you're riding has to stop short, the danger is that the force of the adult's body will be thrown against the child. In such a case, the child could be badly injured.

Car seats are now required in every state for young children, usually under the ages of four or five. Invest in a safe, approved car seat and make sure it is always securely belted to the seat of the automobile. Never simply hold a child in your lap. (For a complete listing of car safety seats approved by consumer experts, consult *The Childwise Catalog: A Consumer Guide to Buying the Safest and Best Products for Your Children,* by Jack Gillis and Mary Ellen R. Fise, Pocket Books, 1985.)

In an airplane, many parents do simply hold children under two in their arms during takeoff and landing, and the airlines condone the practice. This is *not* a safe procedure; studies show that it's impossible to restrain a child in a car or plane during crashes or collisions at speeds greater than thirty miles an hour. Children age two and over are required to wear their own seatbelts on airplanes just like adults. Children under two are best off secured into a special safety seat, like those designed for automobiles.

Since 1982 the Federal Aviation Administration (FAA) has permitted the use of these seats on airplanes. While the individual airlines are not *required* to permit safety seats for infants on board, many of them now do.

If you're going to bring a safety seat on board a plane, make sure it has FAA approval: It must be manufactured more recently than February 26, 1985, and carry two labels: one that states it is "certified for use in motor vehicles and aircraft," and the other stating "This child restraint system conforms to all applicable federal motor vehicle safety standards." Seats manufactured between January 1981 and 1985 are permitted if the label states they conform to federal standards for motor vehicle safety. (The FAA does not permit vests or harness restraints on board aircraft.)

Before you purchase your plane ticket, ask if the airline will permit the safety seat, and check to see if you'll have to purchase a separate ticket for your child. Most airlines *will* require you to buy another seat in this case (although a few will allow a child under two to travel in a safety seat without a ticket if the flight is not full). While it is unfortunately expensive, buying a ticket for your child so he or she can be secured into a safety seat is the smartest, safest way to fly.

TRAVEL COMFORT

On long trips, it's just as important that children take frequent breaks for exercise as it is for adults. For maximum comfort, request bulkhead seats in advance when traveling by air with children. You'll have more room for children to stand up, look out the window, sit on the floor, and play—and fewer neighbors to be annoyed by the noise and activity. If you're trying a stretch or exercise program on board a plane, have your children do it with you if it won't disturb other passengers. At least get up and walk up and down the aisle with them every hour or so.

On long car trips, sacrifice some mileage gains to make sure your children have a twenty minute break to walk, run, and play at least every two hours.

Child-Proofing Your New Environment

Just as having children at home means making adjustments in how you live, so taking children along on a trip requires that you make changes in order to ensure their safety. Whether you're staying in a hotel room, in a cruise ship cabin, or at a friend's house, you should take precautions to eliminate hazards.

Children, especially those between the ages of one and three, tend to put anything they find into their mouths. Check your hotel room—or wherever you're staying—for small objects such as pens, matchbooks, etc., and put them out of harm's way. If you're traveling with drugs, make sure you store them out of sight and out of reach. Buy all medications in child-resistant packages. If there isn't a high enough medicine cabinet in your bathroom, or a high enough shelf in the room, you can also leave medications and any other poisonous substances securely locked in your suitcase. If your room contains a "wet bar" with alcoholic beverages, make sure that the cabinet remains locked and inaccessible to your children. Always obtain the number of the nearest poison control center if you're traveling in the States, and keep it by the telephone. If you're abroad, know how to use the syrup of ipecac you've brought with you in case of accidental poisoning (see chapter 8 for instructions on handling poisoning emergencies), and also know where the nearest emergency room is.

Check the rooms in which you'll be staying for sharp corners on furniture, doors, windows. If you're in a hotel and can't get rid of furniture with sharp edges, you may be able to fit some pieces into corners so that no edges are exposed. If that fails, try covering edges with towels, blankets, or even with heavy tape. Assure yourself that radiators and heating baseboards are concealed behind furniture, and out of children's reach.

Check also for exposed electrical cords that could become wrapped around a child's neck, or on which a child could chew. The most frequent cause of mouth burns in children occurs when youngsters put cords or wires in their mouths. Ideally, plugs and cords from electrical appliances should neither be removable, nor within a child's pulling reach. Make sure there are no frayed or uncovered electrical wires, and that outlets are out of children's reach. If you're traveling in the United States, you can carry safety plugs to cover up unused outlets. If you're abroad, where the outlets are shaped differently than at home, either conceal them with furniture or cover them temporarily with electrical tape.

Finally, assure yourself that windows are out of children's reach, and that there are no chairs, tables, or other furniture on which a child could climb to reach a window. Keep windows locked as much as possible, and don't leave your children unsupervised in the room.

Travelers' Diarrhea

Children, because they are smaller, are at a greater risk for becoming seriously dehydrated from diarrhea than adults are. If you're traveling with infants, it's smartest to bring along either premixed formula or jars of baby food. By keeping young children on their regular diet, you're most likely to prevent stomach problems. Severe diarrhea in infants requires medical attention. Mild diarrhea, however, is probably just a reaction to new food in the diet and a change in routine caused by traveling.

Older children, who will want to be adventurous and sample the local cuisine, should be instructed in how to avoid food and water that may make them sick in countries where turista is a problem. (Young children are less likely to want to try new foods. To appease them, bring along some of their favorite foods from home, such as granola bars, raisins, candy, or cereal—to supplement the unfamiliar food. While you may want to eat bistro food every night on Paris's Left Bank, your children might be happiest with a hamburger from the McDonald's on the Champs Elysées.) To prevent diarrhea and other gastrointestinal illnesses in children, make sure that they follow the same food and water precautions as adults, i.e., only bottled water if the water safety is in question, well-cooked foods, no raw fruits or vegetables that can't be peeled, etc. (See chapter 3 for more specific advice on avoiding travelers' diarrhea.)

Sometimes a child will suffer a case of turista in spite of precautions. Diarrhea is most serious for infants, who can become dehydrated much more quickly than adults and even older children. For the first six to twelve hours, babies should drink small amounts of diluted juices (except apple), water and flat soda instead of cow's milk or formula. But breast-feeding babies should continue breast-feeding. (Milk or formula should be gradually reintroduced after twelve to twenty-four hours.) Children this age can be given Pedialyte, if you've brought it along, but should not drink the homemade rehydration formula (described in chapter 3). Young children should also not take an antimotility drug such as Imodium, or the antibiotic doxycycline (Vibramycin), unless under a physician's orders.

Older infants and toddlers who suffer from turista should drink plenty of fluids and restrict their diet to such soft foods as ripe bananas, rice or rice cereal, applesauce, and toast with jelly.

If your baby or toddler shows no improvement in two days, or if he shows signs of dehydration (dry mouth, listlessness, excessive thirst, sunken eyes), *seek medical attention immediately.* Also consult a doctor if stools turn suddenly loose or watery, if they contain pus or blood, if diarrhea is accompanied by a fever of 101°F. or more, or if diarrhea is accompanied by vomiting.

For older children with diarrhea, bedrest, plenty of fluids (juices, flat carbonated beverages), and foods such as cereals, soups, gelatins, crackers, and bread are the best remedy. Regular foods should be gradually reintroduced as the diarrhea disappears. School-age children can drink Pedialyte or the rehydration formula (described in chapter 3) to prevent dehydration, but children under twelve should not take doxycycline (Vibramycin) unless under a doctor's orders. In general, youngsters should not take any antidiarrhea drugs without a doctor's advice. If there is no improvement in two days, have your child see a physician.

Teenagers with diarrhea should follow the advice for adults, with possible adjustment of medication dosages based on their age and size. See medicine packages for instructions.

Special Precautions in Extreme Heat or Cold

HEAT

Children, for several reasons, are at higher risk for heat injuries than adults are when exercising in hot weather. First, their sweat glands don't work as efficiently as adults' until puberty. Second, they produce more metabolic heat per unit of body mass. Third, their capacity to convey body heat from the internal organs to the skin is lower than adults'. And finally, their ratio of surface area to body weight is higher, forcing them to absorb more heat from the environment.

To protect children from heat injury, such as sun poisoning or heatstroke, make sure that they drink lots of water before and during vigorous exercise. Dress them in loose clothing made of fabrics that "breathe" (such as cotton and some of the newer synthetics designed for athletic wear). When high temperatures are combined with high humidity, don't let your children play outside too hard or too long. Children of all ages, just like adults, should wear a sunscreen when spending time outdoors.

But as anyone who's watched children race around at summer camp knows, most children manage just fine in the heat. Unless your trip is going to be especially hot and strenuous, such as a hike through the Israeli desert, there's no need for any special precautions other than the routine and common sense tips listed above.

COLD

Children, when properly dressed in warm layers of clothing, are at no special risk in cold weather. If they enjoy winter sports such as sledding, skiing, and ice skating on their home turf, there's no reason why they can't enjoy them away from home. And if you and your family reside in a warm climate and are traveling to a cold one, your bodies will signal when it's time to come inside: you'll feel intolerably cold.

Even infants can adapt to almost any temperature as long as they're dressed appropriately. One of the biggest dangers in cold weather is in being too enthusiastic about keeping your child warm. A baby kept in an overheated house or apartment, for example, can develop sniffles or an irritated nose.

This is not to say that you should not be concerned about cold temperatures. For example, infants can develop hypothermia—lowered body temperature—more easily than adults if unprotected and exposed to cold outdoor temperatures, cold water, or underheated rooms for a prolonged time. And while an underdressed baby is at risk of hypothermia, an overbundled infant *can* suffer from heatstroke. Happily, both possibilities occur only at the extreme ends of the spectrum, and are unlikely. (An infant suffering from hypothermia, besides exhibiting the symptoms listed in chapter 6, may also have red cheeks, chin, tip of nose, or limbs. Babies with hypothermia tend to be slower, less alert and less responsive; they also tend not to cry, and to suck weakly when fed. Treatment is the same as for an adult. See chapter 6 for advice on treating hypothermia.)

To protect babies from colds, flu, whooping cough, croup, ear infections, and other illnesses which seem to be most common in cold weather, limit the number of people who have direct contact with your child. When contagious diseases are circulating, the more people who touch your baby, the greater the chance of one of them passing along an illness. Also, if you, your babysitter, and anyone else who comes in contact with the child take care to wash your hands frequently, you are less likely to pass along viruses and other organisms.

Finally, for instructions on how to handle children's emergencies away from home, see chapter 8 on first aid procedures. Of special interest to travelers with children: bites and stings, bleeding (cuts, scrapes, bloody noses), bruises, burns and sunburn, foreign body (in eye, ear, or nose), poisoning, and poison ivy.

11 | Special Travelers, Special Needs

If traveling poses health risks to the hale and hardy, imagine the concerns for people who start out their trips with a health problem or handicap. Even healthy senior citizens must take a few extra precautions. But very few illnesses prevent people from enjoying a vacation these days. Today, even people with health problems that would have limited them to armchair traveling not long ago are enjoying exotic trips to undeveloped areas. Once again, some care and preparation make the difference between a trip fraught with medical peril, and an almost carefree voyage. Remember, the advice in this chapter is designed to be very general. Only your physician knows *your* specific medical history.

Before You Go

The advice on preparing for a trip—in chapter 1—is especially important for elderly travelers or travelers with health problems. A pre-trip physical is crucial, as is consultation with your physician about your itinerary. Arranging for an adequate supply of prescription medication, and checking into vaccinations and other prophylaxis (for malaria, diarrhea, etc.) is essential. Be sure you ask your physician about how time differences will affect your medication doses. Know the generic name of your medication, and the dosage, in case you must replace it while away. Carry your physician's address and phone number with you. It's also smart to learn the name of your illness or condition in the language of your destination. That way, you can at least let a foreign doctor know what you are suffering from in the event of an emergency, or notify him of any allergies to medication.

It's especially important to become an IAMAT or Intermedic member, or to obtain travelers' health insurance before departure (see chapter 1 for more information). In case of a medical emergency, you'll have the name of an English-speaking physician nearby (IAMAT and Intermedic members), or the reassurance of the advice and financial support of an insurance company.

Finally, "special needs" travelers—those with chronic health conditions or handicaps—should carry their medical history with them by obtaining a medical identification device before they depart, if they don't have one already. Medical science has come a long way in recent years, but doctors still can't read minds. So just in case you are ever injured, and are unable to talk (or to communicate with a foreign physician), it's wise to carry something that can communicate with your doctor for you.

A few of the medical identification options:

■ Medic Alert Tags. These tags, which can be worn on a bracelet or necklace, are small metal emblems that are easily visible, and contain two vital pieces of information: the medical condition from which the wearer suffers (for instance, penicillin allergy, cancer, glaucoma, or arthritis) and a toll-free phone number that can be called from anywhere in the world to obtain the wearer's medical history. Medic Alert Tags are most often recommended for people at risk of developing emergency medical problems—diabetics, epileptics, hemophiliacs, for example—but anyone can wear one. The tags, plus lifetime membership, cost $20 each for the basic stainless steel model, $30 each for sterling silver and $38 for gold-filled. For more information:

Medic Alert Foundation
P.O. Box 1009
Turlock, CA 95381
(800) 344-3226. In California call (209) 668-3333.

■ Lens-Card, an emergency medical information card. In this age of plastic credit cards, it seems natural that someone would come up with the idea of making a "credit card" that carries a complete medical history on it. On one end, the card has a small sheet of microfilm with your medical information. On the other end of the card is a small, ten-power magnifying lens—when you bend the card, you can look through the lens and read the microfilm. The card fits easily in a wallet, and comes with stickers that can be placed on your wallet or driver's license to alert emergency help to the presence of the card. The card costs $9.95 plus $1.25 for postage and handling. There is an additional charge of $1.50 for a second sheet of medical information (such as an electrocardiogram). For more information and an application, send a stamped, self-addressed envelope to:

DataVue Products
P.O. Box 3559
Abilene, TX 79604
(915) 698-3712

The American Medical Association (AMA) also offers a medical I.D. card—a simple, old-fashioned wallet card that holds basic medical information. The card is free, from:

AMA
535 North Dearborn Street
Chicago, IL 60610

Medic Alert Tags are probably the most widely recognized medical identification product in the world. If, however, you don't want to *wear* anything, the Lens-Card or AMA card, which fit into your wallet as easily as a credit card, are handy alternatives.

Stress

Even though vacations are supposed to help you relax, they can be fraught with stress—worries about packing what you need, catching the airplane, making connections, fear of flying, and trying to cram every day full of activity so you don't miss anything. And if you're traveling on business . . . well, everything about a business trip is stressful. Almost everybody has experienced stress-related symptoms such as stiff neck, lower back pain, headaches, acne, insomnia, teeth-grinding, and stomach problems. Most people learn to deal successfully with short-term stress, such as travel, when it occurs. But for some people, including those with certain medical conditions, stress can cause more serious problems. Conditions that are aggravated by stress include: angina pectoris, bronchial asthma, hypertension, migraine headaches, and peptic ulcer disease.

To minimize stress's effects on the body, be sure to get plenty of sleep, and try to maintain the same level of exercise and activity as usual (unless factors such as extreme heat, cold, or altitude prevent it). Eating properly and practicing relaxation techniques can also help you minimize and deal with stress.

RELAXATION TECHNIQUES

The following exercise may seem easy and trivial, but the important thing is it works to relieve stress. It's based on the same premise as meditation, but requires no special instruction:

Wearing loose, comfortable clothing, sit down in a comfortable position (don't lie down, because you may fall asleep). Take the phone off the hook. Close your eyes. Breathe deeply. Each time you exhale, concentrate on the number "one." If you find other thoughts intruding, just mentally brush them aside and keep focusing on "one." Do the exercise for ten minutes at a time.

When you're feeling very stressed and don't have the opportunity to practice the relaxation exercise—for instance, when you're stuck in the middle of a traffic jam—breathe deeply to calm yourself. Also, you can alternately tense and release your muscles, starting with your toes and continuing up to your neck and forehead, to relax. Listening to soothing music may also help.

Airplane Alerts

Flying poses special hazards for people with health problems. Even though airplane cabins are pressurized, they contain only about 80 percent of the oxygen at sea level—equivalent to an altitude of about 7,000 feet. While this difference is barely noticed by most travelers, people with asthma, emphysema, and other lung disorders, angina pectoris, and other heart or circulatory problems, may have difficulty. The standard rule for determining if someone is able to fly is that if he's able to walk a block or climb a flight of stairs without stopping or becoming short of breath, he'll be okay on an airplane. Anyone in doubt should check with a physician before booking a flight. A doctor may recommend that some people contact the airline in advance and request that they provide extra oxygen, just in case. The airline will need a physician's prescription for the amount of oxygen required. (Patients cannot bring their own oxygen tanks on board commercial aircraft.)

Post-surgery and heart attack or stroke patients should wait until their physicians consider it safe for them to fly. Doctors usually recommend that airplane travel be avoided for a month after a heart attack, and for at least two weeks after a stroke, or after eye, chest, or abdominal surgery.

Others who should avoid flying or consult a doctor first: people with severe anemia or other blood disorders, women with high-risk pregnancies, or women past the eighth month of pregnancy.

Air pressure differences mean that colostomy patients should use a bag one size larger than usual during long flights (four hours or longer). Also, colostomy patients who clean the stoma with ether should make other arrangements for on board the plane. Ether is highly flammable, and is dangerous on an aircraft, especially when there is smoking on board. Very few stoma patients still use ether, but those who do should find a substitute cleanser for airplane travel.

Migraine sufferers may find that plane travel—and any greater-than-usual altitude—brings on an attack. They should carry necessary medication on board just in case.

People with glaucoma should check with their doctors to make sure that the altered airplane pressure will not affect the pressure in their eyes.

Travelers with pacemakers, artificial joints, or shrapnel (from war injuries) in their bodies should carry a note from their physician, since they will probably set off airport metal detectors each time they walk through them.

For comfort's sake, anyone with a bad cold or acute upper respiratory infection, sinus problem, or nasal polyps should avoid flying until the condition has cleared up or been treated. Likewise for people with dental cavities or periodontal abscesses. It's also a good idea to avoid flying for at least forty-eight hours after any dental procedure, to avoid pain due to the altered cabin pressure.

Many commercial airlines can, given twenty-four hours' notice, provide meals to accommodate special diets, such as low-sodium, salt-free, low-caloric, low-carbohydrate, diabetic, low-fat, bland, low-cholesterol, high-protein, gluten-free, hypoglycemic, or lactose-restricted. (Cruise ships can also usually arrange to accommodate special diets.) If you are on a special diet and the airline you're flying can't provide the proper diet, you'll probably have to bring your own food on board.

Wheelchair-bound passengers must give the airline forty-eight hours' notice to have an attendant waiting with a special chair that can fit down a plane's narrow aisles. Usually, passengers in wheelchairs must be accompanied by a person familiar with their medical problem. British Airways has recently introduced a wheelchair with a removable armrest and back on its transatlantic flights (all 747 and L-1011 planes); the chair allows disabled travelers to get to the restrooms themselves. United Airlines has a wheelchair on board each of its 767s and most of its DC8-71s, as well as restrooms with connecting doors that face each other and can be locked open to provide wheelchair-bound passengers with privacy and maneuverability.

Blind and deaf persons should identify themselves to airline personnel after boarding, so that they can be kept informed of all safety procedures and announcements. Blind people with guide dogs should check before leaving to make sure that their dogs will be allowed to accompany them in the airplane cabin. Most, but not all, airlines allow guide dogs to travel at the feet of their owners. Also check in advance with the embassy of the country you'll be visiting, since some will not permit guide dogs to enter, or require a six month quarantine period; these countries include Australia, Hong Kong, Ireland, New Zealand, the United Kingdom (and British Islands in the Caribbean), and the state of Hawaii. Some countries, such as Sweden, Norway, and Denmark (and Caribbean islands which are part of the Netherlands), require a certificate that the dog has been recently vaccinated against rabies. You must check the specific regulations before you depart, or you and your dog may be refused entrance into a country, or your dog may be held in quarantine for months.

Travelers' Diarrhea

Simple turista can be a serious problem for people with certain illnesses. Dehydration due to excessive fluid loss, such as that caused by diarrhea, can exacerbate such illnesses as heart disease, diabetes, and kidney disease. People with these conditions should ask their doctor about taking prophylactic antibiotics to reduce their chances of picking up an intestinal bug. Also, people taking anti-ulcer medication such as cimetidine (Tagamet), ranitidine (Zantac), or antacids, should also see about taking prophylactic antibiotics. Doctors have found that these anti-ulcer drugs make turista more likely.

Special Advice for People with Serious Health Problems

CANCER

Traveling for cancer patients is a very individual thing. Most people in remission have no restrictions on their travel. But even people undergoing radiation or chemotherapy (on an outpatient basis) can travel. Your physician may say that you can skip therapy for the duration for a trip, or he may make arrangements with a doctor or cancer center abroad to continue your therapy while you are away. For a listing of cancer centers around the world, see either *The Cancer Reference Book* (By Paul M. Levitt and Elissa S. Guralnick et al., Facts on File, New York, 1979, 1983), or contact *COPE* (a magazine for cancer patients) at: Suite B400, 12600 West Colfax Avenue, Denver, CO 80215. The publisher of *COPE* also publishes a book called *Cancer World*, International Travel Guide and Glossary for Cancer Patients, which subscribers to *COPE* receive for free.

Patients on radiation or chemotherapy, whose immune systems are compromised by the treatment, should check into supplemental vaccines such as the pneumococcal vaccine.

DIABETES

Diabetics must deal both with dietary challenges and with changes in medication schedules when they travel. Anyone with diabetes who has been able to manage restaurant meals and business lunches successfully should be able to continue their vigilance on a vacation. To be safe, it's smart for diabetics to carry their own food (such as cheese, crackers, juice, fruit, raisins, nuts, candy bars) on board planes and at all other times, for both quick and slow sources of carbohydrates, and so that no meals have to be skipped.

Jet lag and time changes pose a challenge to people who receive insulin injections (tablets are usually not affected). Check with your doctor about altering your insulin schedule if you're crossing several time zones, even if your insulin is taken in twenty-four hour doses. (Also check with a physician if you would like to follow the anti-jet lag diet, described in chapter 2.) When planning your insulin schedule, a good general rule to follow is: Keep your watch set to your home time while you are on board the plane, and follow your usual eating schedule (you can arrange with the airline in advance for a diabetic meal, and you can request that the meal be served at a specific time). Then, when you arrive at your destination, adjust your watch to the new time, and adjust your next dose of insulin per your physician's instructions. In general, if your day is shorter because you've flown from west to east, you will have to reduce the dose slightly. If the day is longer because you've flown west, you should increase the dose slightly.

An altered eating schedule, motion sickness, heat exhaustion, and diarrhea can interfere with sugar control. Stick to your diet, maintain your weight, and check blood and urine sugar levels frequently as you travel.

Insulin travels well and remains potent for three months, but it shouldn't be kept too cold (for instance, in the baggage compartment of a plane) or too hot (in the trunk of a car, for example). If you must buy insulin abroad, you'll probably have to see a doctor, since it is sold by prescription only in most countries. Make sure that you receive the correct dosage, since U-100, the insulin most Americans use, is not always available abroad. If overzealous customs or border agents confiscate your syringes, you can usually replace them in a local pharmacy. To be safe, carry a note from your doctor describing your condition.

Other precautions: Avoid excessive sun exposure and sunburn, check with your physician about having the pneumococcal vaccine, and be very diligent about foot and skin care, since blisters and scratches can start serious infections.

For more information, you can write for several free booklets. "Vacations, Travel, and Diabetes" is available from Becton Dickinson Consumer Products, P.O. Box 5000, Rochelle Park, NJ 07662; the phone number is (800) 237-4554. You can also write for the booklet, "Traveling with Diabetes" from: Squibb-Novo, P.O. Box 4000, Princeton, NJ 08543-4000. The American Diabetes Association can also provide information about traveling; the address is 1660 Duke Street, Alexandria, VA 22314. Finally, for a list of diabetes specialists around the world, write to International Diabetes Federation, 40 Washington Street, 1050 Brussels, Belgium.

HEART DISEASE

Doctors now believe that it is safe for most cardiac patients to travel . . . with a few caveats. Carry a copy of your most recent ECG (electrocardiogram) in case you require medical attention while away. Extreme heat or altitude (over five thousand feet) should be avoided, unless your physician gives you the okay. Heart patients should also ask about having the pneumococcal vaccine, since pneumonia can be especially serious for them. Hypertensives or others on a low-sodium diet should be wary of bottled mineral waters, since some contain unacceptably high levels of salt.

Patients with angina pectoris, a condition in which the heart is deprived of oxygen during exertion, excitement, or cold, will have to be careful not to let the stress of traveling affect the condition (doctors have even coined the term "airport angina" to describe angina pain brought on by rushing for an airplane, carrying luggage, etc.).

People taking anticoagulant medication, who must have their blood-clotting mechanism measured regularly to determine the proper dosage of medication, can also travel. Laboratories in major cities around the world perform this test, and your physician can make arrangements for you in advance.

Individuals with pacemakers should have the batteries tested before the voyage to make sure they will last the duration. Carry medical records which show the name of the manufacturer, the type of pacemaker, the model number, type of electrode, and date of implantation.

This information will help if a foreign doctor must examine you while you are away. Also, carry the phone number of the cardiologist or doctor who regularly checks your pacemaker, since it can be checked as you travel either by a local hospital, or by long-distance telephone to your own doctor or clinic.

Traveling companions of people who have had a heart attack, or of people who are considered at high risk (people with high blood pressure, for example), should take a course in cardiopulmonary resuscitation (CPR). When medical help isn't immediately available, knowing CPR can save lives.

Contact your local American Heart Association for more information.

KIDNEY DISEASE

Even dialysis patients can travel, if arrangements for continuing treatment are made in advance. For a list of dialysis facilities worldwide, contact the National Association of Patients on Hemodialysis and Transplantation, 150 Nassau Street, New York, NY 10038. Telephone: (212) 619-2727.

LUNG AND RESPIRATORY DISEASES (INCLUDING ASTHMA, BRONCHITIS, EMPHYSEMA, ETC.)

Altitude, oxygen, and allergens are the primary concerns of patients with respiratory diseases. At altitudes over five thousand feet such as in Mexico City, Nairobi, or Denver, some people may get short of breath, or require supplemental oxygen. Check with your doctor before you leave to see if your destination's altitude could pose a problem. Exercise, weather changes (cold, rain, humidity), and pollution (for instance, in cities such as Los Angeles or Tokyo) can also cause breathing problems for asthmatics or people with bronchitis; be prepared for a worsening of symptoms in these instances. A new environment can also mean newly discovered allergies for some asthma patients. Again, be prepared with medication. Anyone suffering from respiratory disease should ask their physicians about the pneumococcal vaccine, since pneumonia could be particularly dangerous for them.

The Handicapped

For handicapped persons, the primary travel concern is access. Will you be able to use airplanes, buses, trains? Will you be able to enter hotels, museums, restaurants? The international symbol of accessibility is an outline of a person in a wheelchair. Airlines, train and bus companies, hotels, and tourist offices can often provide a great deal of information. Also, there are now numerous resources and guides which address the concerns of wheelchair-bound and disabled travelers. A few:

BOOKS AND NEWSLETTERS

Access to the World (A Travel Guide for the Handicapped), by Louise Weiss, Facts on File, 1983.

Frommer's Guide for the Disabled Traveler: United States, Canada and Europe, by Frances Barish, Simon & Schuster, 1984.

LTD Travel, a four-times-a-year newsletter that covers destinations and their accessibility, as well as news, travel tips, itineraries, and book reviews. A one-year subscription costs $15, and is available from: LTD Travel, 116 Harbor Seal Court, San Mateo, CA 94404. Phone number: (415) 573-7998.

ORGANIZATIONS THAT CAN PROVIDE INFORMATION

Society for the Advancement of Travel for the Handicapped
26 Court Street
Brooklyn, NY 11242
(718) 858-5483

Travel Information Service
Moss Rehabilitation Hospital
12th Street and Tabor Road
Philadelphia, PA 19141
(215) 329-5715

Rehabilitation International USA
1123 Broadway
Suite 704
New York, NY 10001
(publishes an International Directory of Access Guides, available for $10)

Airport Operators Council International, Inc.
1220 19th Street N.W.
Suite 800
Washington, D.C. 20036
(202) 293-8500
(publishes "Access Travel: A Guide to Accessibility of Airport Terminals")

SPECIAL TOURS AND CRUISES

For the deaf:
Ruth Skinner's Interpret Tours
Encino Travel Service, Inc.
16660 Ventura Boulevard
Encino, CA 91436
(818) 788-4118

FOR THE HANDICAPPED

Whole Person Tours
P.O. Box 1084
Bayonne, NJ 07002
(201) 858-3400
(also publishes a magazine, "The Itinerary," with information for handicapped travelers; the magazine is published six times a year, and costs $7 for a one-year subscription)

Flying Wheels Tours
143 West Bridge Street
Box 382
Owatonna, MN 55060
(800) 533-0363 (in Minnesota call (507) 451-5005)

Evergreen Travel Service
19505 44th Avenue West
Lynnwood, WA 98306
(206) 776-1184
(organizes luxury tours overseas for the handicapped)

The Elderly

Even healthy elderly people should take some extra precautions to ensure that they return home at least as healthy as they left. A pre-trip physical exam is essential, and at that time the patient and doctor should discuss immunization, diarrhea prophylaxis, and any other recommended precautions. Besides the usual recommended vaccines, senior citizens should ask their doctor about the pneumococcal and influenza vaccines or prophylactic drugs. Older individuals should *never* travel without health insurance. For more information, including special health insurance for senior citizens provided by the American Association of Retired Persons, see chapter 1.

Fatigue is one of the biggest problems for older travelers, who should be certain to plan plenty of relaxation time into their itineraries. Elderly people are also more likely to be adversely affected by environmental conditions than younger travelers. Heatstroke and hypothermia, due to excessive heat or cold, are much more likely to occur in older people. Older cardiovascular systems may not operate as efficiently as younger ones to regulate body temperature, so a lesser degree of heat or cold can pose a threat. In addition, senior citizens are more likely to be taking medication, which can also affect the body's thermostat. High altitudes, too, may be difficult for older people to tolerate. Make sure your physician knows your itinerary, as well as all the medications you will be traveling with (drug side effects and drug interactions can sometimes be a problem for older voyagers who regularly take several medications, then add several more on a trip to prevent turista or malaria). And see chapter 6 for precautions against environmental illnesses.

12 | When You Need Help

Of the one in three travelers who become ill abroad, most will not require medical attention, since the 33 percent includes such minor complaints as colds, flu, and diarrhea. A quick dip into the travelers' medical kit, or, if necessary, a foray to the local pharmacy, should take care of the majority of complaints.

But when more serious illness strikes and travelers need a medical professional, they are often bewildered by the prospect of seeking qualified care. Even in a real emergency, when a patient is rushed to the nearest medical facility, there will eventually be choices to make, such as whether to complete the treatment in a foreign hospital once the emergency is past, or to fly back home for care. Last year, nearly one million American travelers required medical attention overseas.

Some people have taken steps before traveling so that they are prepared for a medical crisis. IAMAT and Intermedic members (see chapter 1) have a list of English-speaking doctors around the world who will see them for a modest fee. And people with travel insurance usually have access to a hotline that can dispense advice and recommend English-speaking physicians.

If, however, you hoped for the best and didn't make arrangements in advance to deal with medical problems, you will have to use the resources around you to ensure you get good health care. The following advice on shopping in a foreign pharmacy, choosing a foreign physician, and dealing with foreign hospitalization, can help you be a good medical consumer, no matter where you are. Finally, the chapter ends with a list of helpful phrases pertaining to health, and their translations into nine languages.

Drugs and Drugstores: What's Over-the-Counter? What's Prescription? Plus Shopping in a Foreign Pharmacy

Many medical experts divide the world into two parts according to the prevailing attitude on drugs. On the one side are the United States, England and the United Kingdom, Scandinavia, and the Netherlands: These nations exert rather stringent control over the sale of drugs.

On the other side are central and southern Europe, Asia, Africa, Central and South America: These countries sell most medications without prescriptions, or over-the-counter. *Don't* make the mistake of thinking that just because a drug is available without a prescription it is not very strong, and is perfectly safe. Very powerful drugs are sold over-the-counter in much of the world.

Americans have the security of knowing that the Food and Drug Administration (FDA) exerts strict controls over the sale and quality of drugs in this country. But Americans must be very careful about buying medications abroad. Many drugs sold overseas are not available in the United States, because they were not found to be "safe and effective" by the FDA. One example is a drug called aminopyrine (Piramidon), for colds and headaches. Sold in Italy and much of Europe, this drug was banned in the U.S. in 1938 after it was discovered that it can destroy the blood's white cells, and can even be fatal.

Other drugs either banned in the U.S. or not approved by the FDA for the conditions they are used for abroad include:

■ Chloramphenicol, for treating colds and diarrhea. Because one of its side effects is the risk of bone marrow depression and aplastic anemia, this medication is used in the U.S. only for the treatment of diseases such as typhoid fever, H. influenzae, typhus, plague, and Rocky Mountain spotted fever . . . and then it is usually administered in a hospital, after frequent blood tests. But if you come down with a case of travelers' diarrhea abroad, this drug may be offered to you over-the-counter.

■ Iodochlorhydroxyquin (brand names Enterovioform and Mexaform), for preventing diarrhea. The sale of this drug has been prohibited in the United States since 1971, because it is considered ineffective and dangerous (one of its possible side effects is blindness).

Ideally, of course, travelers will never have to make medical purchases. If you take along a travelers' medical kit and extra supplies of your prescription drugs, chances are you won't need to venture into a foreign pharmacy at all.

But should the need ever arise, you are best off with medications with which you are comfortable and familiar—the same medications you take at home. You can shop for familiar medications in several ways:

■ If you have the empty packet of your medication, bring it into the pharmacy with you, show it to the pharmacist, and ask him for the same medicine in the same dosage. He should recognize the generic name, and perhaps even the manufacturer, and be able to supply you with an equivalent. (If you lose or run out of your prescription medication, you can always try a local pharmacy to see if they will sell you the equivalent drug over-the-counter before you make an appointment with a foreign doctor to obtain a prescription.)

■ If you don't have the medicine container, but remember the generic name, you may be able to replace the medicine with its equivalent that way. The pharmacist should recognize the generic name.

In many cases, the exact drug to which you're accustomed, manufactured by the same company, will be available, sometimes even under the same name. In other cases, the same medication will simply be in an unfamiliar package, and be sold under a different brand name.

If you find yourself with a splitting headache, a runny nose, or a queasy stomach, and have no idea what to ask for, the following is a list of some common over-the-counter medications for travel ailments, and their foreign equivalents:

GENERIC NAME: acetaminophen (also called paracetamol)
BRAND NAMES IN U.S.: Anacin-3, Datril, Panadol, Tylenol, St. Joseph Aspirin-Free for Children, and others
USED TO TREAT: Pain (including headaches, muscle aches, menstrual cramps), fever
BRAND NAMES ABROAD: Dozens of different names. Best simply to ask for acetaminophen or paracetamol.

GENERIC NAME: diphenhydramine
BRAND NAMES IN U.S.: Benadryl, Benylin, Compōz, Nytol, Sominex, and others
USED TO TREAT: Allergies, coughs, insomnia, motion sickness

BRAND NAMES ABROAD:
United Kingdom: Benadryl, Benafed, Benylin, Guanor, Histalix, Histergan, Lotussin, Ticipect
Australia: Alergicap, Bidramine
Canada: Insomnal, Somnium
Denmark: Amidryl
Germany: Dolestan, Halbmond, Pheramin
Italy: Allergan, Allergina, Dermistina
South Africa: Dihydral
Spain: Teldrin
Sweden: Desentol
Switzerland: Benocten, Cathejell, Dobacen, Felben, Neo-Synodorm, Somenox

GENERIC NAME: ibuprofen
BRAND NAMES IN U.S.: Advil, Nuprin, Motrin (by prescription only), Rufen (by prescription only)
USED TO TREAT: Pain, including menstrual cramps, arthritis, tendinitis, bursitis, and other inflammatory diseases
BRAND NAMES ABROAD:
United Kingdom (plus Australia, Belgium, Denmark, France, Germany, Italy, Japan, Netherlands, Norway, South Africa, Spain, Sweden, Switzerland): Brufen, Ebufac, Ibu-Slo
Argentina: Emodin
Australia: Inflam
Canada: Amersol, Motrin
Italy: Algofen, Focus, Rebugen
Japan: Andran, Anflagen, Bluton, Brufanic, Donjust B, Epobron, IB-100, Ibuprocin, Lamidon, Liptan, Mynosedin, Nagifen-D, Napacetin, Nobfelon, Nobgen, Pantrop, Roidenin
South Africa: Inza

GENERIC NAME: kaolin
BRAND NAME IN U.S.: Kaopectate
USED TO TREAT: Diarrhea
BRAND NAMES ABROAD: Kaopectate, Kaylene, KLN Suspension (for children)

GENERIC NAME: meclizine
BRAND NAMES IN U.S.: Bonine, Antivert (by prescription only)
USED TO TREAT: Motion sickness
BRAND NAMES ABROAD:
United Kingdom: Ancoloxin
Argentina: Bonamina

Australia: Ancolan
Belgium: Postafene
Canada: Bonamine
Denmark: Postafen
Germany: Bonamine, Calmonal, Peremesin, Postafen
Italy: Neo-Isfafene
Netherlands: Postafene, Suprimal
Norway: Postafen
South Africa: Navicalm
Spain: Chiclida, Navicalm, Supermesin
Sweden: Postafen
Switzerland: Duremesan, Peremesin

GENERIC NAME: Pseudoephedrine
BRAND NAMES IN U.S.: Actifed, Afrinol Repetabs, Congestac, Dimacol, Drix-
oral, Fedrazil, Sine-Aid, Sinutab, Sudafed, and others
USED TO TREAT: Colds, allergies, upper respiratory infections, nasal congestion
BRAND NAMES ABROAD:
  United Kingdom: Actifed, Extil, Linctifed, Paragesic, Sudafed
  Australia: Droxora Repetabs, Sudelix
  Brazil: Isofedrin
  Canada: Eltor, Robidrine

If the medication you're looking for isn't on this list, a clinic in California runs a phone-line called the Medication Information Service to provide foreign drug equivalents over the phone. You can call from anywhere in the world (although it's smarter to call before you travel). Give the pharmacist the name of your medication, and the names of the countries you'll be visiting, and he'll give you the trade names of your medicine at your destinations. The number is: (213) 376-3000; in California, call (800) 255-DRUG.

Before you take a medication that you've purchased abroad, check the dosage carefully. You may take two tablets of 200 mg. each at home, but the tablets you buy abroad might contain 300 mg. of medication. In that case, you should only take a tablet and a half, rather than two tablets, to get the same amount of medicine.

Also, you may have noticed that aspirin is missing from the list above. That is because in spite of the many brand names it is sold under in this country and abroad, the word for "aspirin" (which is the generic name in the U.S. and most countries, but a trademark in some) is pretty universal. For instance, in Spanish the drug is called "aspirina." If you walk into a drugstore and ask for aspirin (or acetylsalicylic acid, which is also its generic name), you shouldn't have any trouble finding what you want.

Is There a Doctor in the House?

When you or someone you are traveling with is in the midst of a true medical emergency, you won't have the opportunity to be too specific about who your doctor is or what the hospital's reputation is, since time is of the essence. Many Americans tend to underestimate the severity of their medical problems, and not seek medical care quickly enough. While certain symptoms—such as bleeding and broken bones—always bring a patient to the emergency room, other less dramatic symptoms that require immediate treatment may be overlooked. As a guide to seeking emergency treatment, the American College of Emergency Physicians lists these seven warning signs of a medical emergency:

1). Chest or upper abdominal pain or pressure (a heart attack is frequently mistaken for indigestion).
2). Difficulty in breathing or shortness of breath.
3). Fainting or feeling faint.
4). Dizziness, sudden weakness, or a severe change in vision.
5). Sudden severe pain anywhere in the body.
6). Severe or persistent vomiting.
7). Suicidal or homicidal feelings.

In any of these instances, it's important to contact a physician as soon as possible.

Also, don't ignore these other important symptoms: a fever over 101° F. (38.3°C.) that lasts for two or more days; shaking chills; a persistent stiff neck; diarrhea or abdominal pain lasting more than two or three days; urinary or fecal retention; poisoning, including animal or snake bites.

In any of these instances, it's important to contact a physician as soon as possible. These symptoms could indicate a variety of illnesses much more severe than run-of-the-mill travelers' viruses and stomach problems. In order to rule out serious disease—or confirm illness and begin treatment—you must seek medical care as soon as possible.

Assuming your symptoms do not indicate a real emergency, take a few moments to make sure you really need a doctor before you spend a lot of time and effort to find one. The easiest and most reassuring way to do this is simple: Call your doctor at home. For the price of a long-distance phone call, you can save yourself a lot of worry and a foreign fortune in medical bills. And you get the advice of someone you trust on whether that burning in your stomach is really the beginning of an ulcer, or whether it's just the spicy chili you ate the previous night.

Once it's determined that you really should see a doctor, the best sources for information are your hotel plus the American consulate. (The consulate, which provides services for American citizens abroad, is always part of the embassy. But, while each foreign country has only one embassy, it may have several consulates, located in major cities.)

Most hotels keep the names of doctors who have agreed to pay "house calls" to guests in their hotel rooms. Make sure the doctor speaks English, or that someone from the hotel will be present to translate. If the hotel is reputable and reliable, the doctor probably will be, too.

The American consulate can also provide you with the names of English-speaking physicians. They maintain lists of doctors they consider competent, with information on their specialties, and whether or not they speak English. (When there is no American consulate nearby, the staffs at the consulates of Canada, Great Britain, or Australia may be helpful.)

If necessary, the consulate will also call the States for you to let family and friends know your condition. Finally, they can help arrange transportation back to the U.S. for the seriously ill—and will even provide an escort if necessary. But all costs—doctor bills, hospitalization, transportation, and so forth—must be paid by the patient.

When you first arrive in a foreign country, you should jot down the phone numbers of the consulate—most have a number for regular business hours, and an emergency number where a staff member can be reached nights or holidays. Carry these numbers with you at all times.

If none of these avenues is available to you, because there are no tourist facilities or American consulates in the city you are visiting, or because you are traveling in a rural area, go to the nearest university hospital. The universal sign for hospital is a white "H" on a blue background . . . even in countries where the word for hospital doesn't begin with an "h." If you can't find a university hospital, and your medical situation isn't an emergency, head for the closest big city for care.

When You Require Hospitalization

Americans hospitalized abroad are often frightened by the differences they perceive. In Italy, for instance, some small hospitals require that their patients bring their own linens and food. In Japan, the doctors' manners toward their patients are extremely overbearing and abrupt. Some foreign hospitals may be in antiquated buildings with peeling paint, bare light bulbs, and old furniture. Don't judge the quality of foreign medical care by the surroundings. American hospitals tend to look newer and more comfortable than European or other foreign counterparts, but the building's age has little to do with the quality of the care you'll receive inside. Also, doctors' manners toward their patients vary from nation to nation. Americans are among the most knowledgeable medical consumers in the world, so their physicians offer more information and explanation. Foreign doctors can be much more paternalistic, even autocratic. But a physician's off-putting manner does not indicate lack of knowledge or inadequate medical training. It's important to remember that superficial differences like these reflect differences in customs, and do not necessarily mean that the medical care is incompetent. And remember that a local doctor may be best at diagnosing a local disease, such as a parasitic infection.

Judging the quality of the medical care you receive abroad is difficult, since unless you are a physician or health care professional yourself, you rely on what the doctor tells you for information.

To reassure yourself that you are receiving proper treatment, again, call your doctor in the States. Tell him what your symptoms are, what the diagnosis is, and what medications you are receiving (know the generic rather than the brand name of any drugs, since the brand names can differ from country to country). Make sure your physician is aware of your travel itinerary, so that he can keep "local" diseases in mind when diagnosing you. Ask your doctor, and ask at the consulate, what the country's general medical reputation is, and whether there are any world-renowned medical centers nearby in which you could be treated.

But keep in mind that it's not necessary to receive the world's top medical care for a routine problem such as a broken bone or appendicitis. A good hospital just about anywhere in the world can care for these problems adequately. But if you require delicate, risky, or unusual surgery, or are suffering from a rare ailment, you should assess your options very carefully. If it's possible for you to be moved safely, there are "air ambulances," with medical personnel and equipment on board, which can evacuate you to the States. But these services are *very* expensive. Depending on how far you're traveling and how much medical care you require on board (stretcher, oxygen, doctor, etc.), the cost can range from just a few thousand to over fifty thousand dollars. (Most travelers' health insurance policies—see chapter 1—will cover the cost of emergency evacuation home when they've satisfied themselves that it's truly necessary.) Many people feel it's worth it to be flown home, where they can understand their doctors, and where they have the support of their family and friends. Make the decision carefully, because a lot of unnecessary money is spent flying people back to America, when they could have been treated just as well, and much more economically, by staying put.

Whether you decide to complete your treatment in a foreign hospital, or opt for evacuation home, the American consulate can help you make the arrangements and inform your friends and relatives of your condition (assuming you don't have travel insurance that will take care of these things for you). Before you leave home, you should make sure that your friends and relatives have the State Department's special number in Washington, D.C. where they can call for information on your medical status and help you arrange medical evacuation. The number is (202) 647-5225; nights, weekends, and in real emergencies call (202) 647-1512 or (202) 634-3600.

Breaking the Language Barrier

When travelers are confronted with a health problem abroad, one of the most frightening elements is the difficulty of communicating what's wrong. When you cannot make yourself understood, or understand those around you, even walking into a drugstore for allergy medicine can be an ordeal: You can't ask for what you want; you can't tell the pharmacist what's wrong; you can't even find what you need on the shelf. And since you're not feeling well to begin with, it becomes doubly trying. The situation is even more fraught with terror if you become sick enough to need a foreign doctor, or be taken to a foreign emergency room, where no one speaks English. Not being able to describe your symptoms or tell anyone what is happening can make even the most level-headed individuals panic.

To put you a bit more in control of your health care when traveling, the following is a chart of some simple phrases, translated into nine different languages, which may help you communicate with a foreign doctor or pharmacist:

FRENCH
1. I'd like something for . . . a cold / a cough / constipation / diarrhea / flu / headache / insect bites.

J'aimerais quelque chose contre . . . le rhume / la toux / la constipation / la diarrhée / la grippe / le mal de tête / les piqûres d'insectes.

(zhehmerray kehlkershoze kawntre . . . ler room / lah too / lah constepah-see-on / lah dee-ah-reh / lah mal de tet / lay peek-oor dansect)

2. I take this medicine regularly. (show the medicine)

   Je prends ce médicament régulièrement.

   (zher prahn sir meh-deekah-mahn rehgool-yar-mahn)

3. Can you get me a doctor?

   Pourriez-vous m'appeler un médecin?

   (poor-ree-ay voo mahperlay ang maydssang)

4. Call an ambulance.

   Appelez une ambulance.

   (ahperlay ewn ahnbewlahnss)

5. I have a pain here. (point to the spot)

   J'ai mal ici.

   (zhay mal ee-see)

SPANISH

1. I'd like something for . . . a cold / a cough / constipation / diarrhea / flu / headache / insect bites.

   Desearía algo para . . . el catarro / la tos / el estreñimiento / la diarrea / la gripe / dolor de cabeza / las picaduras.

   (daysayahreeah algo para . . . el catarro / lah toss / el estrenyeemee-ento / lah dee-ah-reh-ah / la greep-eh / doelor deh cahbaytha / las pikadooras)

2. I take this medicine regularly. (show the medicine)

   Tomo esta medicina regularmente.

   (tomo esta meditheena regoolarmenteh)

3. Can you get me a doctor?

   ¿Puede usted buscarme un médico?

   (pwayday oostayd booskahrmay oon maydeekoe)

4. Call an ambulance.

   Llame a una ambulancia.

   Lyahmay ah oonah ahmboolahnthyah)

5. I have a pain here. (point to the spot)

   Tengo un dolor aquí.

   (tayngoe oon doelor ahkee)

GERMAN

1. I'd like something for . . . a cold / a cough / constipation / diarrhea /
   flu / headache / insect bites.

   *Ich möchte etwas gegen . . . Erkältung / Husten / Verstopfung /
   Durchfall / Grippe / Kopfschmerzen / Insektenstiche.*

   (ikh murkhter ehtvahss gaygern . . . erkeltoong / hoosten / fershtop-
   foong / doorshfahl / grippeh / kopfshmayrtzen / inzektenshteesheh)

2. I take this medicine regularly. (show the medicine)

   Ich nehme regelmässig dieses Medikament.

   (ish naymeh raigellmassik deezes medikament)

3. Can you get me a doctor?

   Können Sie einen Arzt für mich finden?

   (kurnen zee eyenern ahrts fewr mikh findern)

4. Call an ambulance.

   Rufen Sie einen Krankenwagen.

   (roofen zee eyenern krahngkernvargern)

5. I have a pain here. (point to the spot)

   Ich habe hier Schmerzen.

   (ich hahbeh here schmayrtzen)

ITALIAN

1. I'd like something for . . . a cold / a cough / constipation / diarrhea / flu / headache / insect bites.

   Vorrei qualcosa per . . . il raffreddore / la tosse / stitichezza / diarrea / influenza / mal di testa / punture di'insetto.

   (vorrayee kwahlkawssah pair . . . eel rahffraydoaray / lah toassay / stitikettza / dee-ahreh-ah / influentza / mal dee testah / poontooreh dansettoh)

2. I take this medicine regularly. (show the medicine)

   Prendo regolarmente questa medicina.

   (prendo regolarmenteh questa medicheena)

3. Please call a doctor.

   Chiamate un medico, per favore.

   (keeahmahtay oon maydeekoh, pair fahvohray)

4. Call an ambulance.

   Chiamate un ambulanza.

   (keeahmahtay oon ahmboolahntsah)

5. I have a pain here. (point to the place)

   Ho un dolore qui.

   (oh oon doloreh kwee)

PORTUGUESE

1. I'd like something for . . . a cold / a cough / constipation / diarrhea / flu / headache / insect bites.

   Queria qualquer coisa para . . . resfriado / tosse / constipação / diarreia / gripe / dor de cabeça / mordidelas de inseto.

   (kerree-ah kwahlkehr coyza para . . . rehfree-ahjo / toss / con-shteepassown / dee-arraya / greep / dor de cabaytha / moordeede-lash dansetto)

2. I take this medicine regularly. (Show the medicine)

   Tomo este medicamento regularmente.

   (tomoo esht medeecamentoo regoolarment)

3. Can you get me a doctor?

   Pode chamar-me um médico?

   (podher shermahr-mer oong medeekoo)

4. Call an ambulance.

   Chame uma ambulância.

   (shermer oomah ermboolahngseer)

5. I have a pain here. (point to the spot)

   Tenho uma dor aqui.

   (tainyoo oomah dor akee)

CHINESE
1. I'd like something for . . . a cold / a cough / constipation / diarrhea /
   flu / headache / insect bites.

   我需要一点药治···感冒···咳嗽···大便干燥··· 痢疾···流感··

   头痛···虫咬。

   Wǒ xū yaò yi diǎn yaò zhì . . . gǎn mào / ké sòu / dà biàn gān zào / lì jí
   / líu gǎn / tóu tòng / chóng yǎo.

2. I take this medicine regularly. (show the medicine)

   我经常使用这种药。

   Wǒ jìng cháng shǐ yòng zhè zhǒng yào.

3. Can you get me a doctor?

请您帮我找一下医生。

Chǐng nín bāng wǒ zhǎo yī xìa yī shēng.

4. Call an ambulance.

请您叫一下救护车。

Chǐng nín jiào yī xìa jìu hù chē.

5. I have a pain here. (point to the spot)

我这里有点痛。

Wǒ zhè lǐ yoú diǎn tòng.

JAPANESE

1. Please give me some . . . medicine

　かぜのお薬を下さい。

　a. Kaze no okusuri o kudasai /cold

　せきのお薬を下さい。

　b. Seki no okusuri o kadusai /cough

　便秘のお薬を下さい。

　c. Benpi no okusuri o kudasai /constipation

　下痢のお薬を下さい。

　d. Geri no okusuri o kudasai /diarrhea

　頭痛のお薬を下さい。

　e. Zutsuu no okusuri o kudasai /headache

刺されたときに使うお薬を下さい。

  f. Sasaretta toki ni tsukau o kusuri o kudasai / insect bites

2. I take this medicine regularly.

私はこのお薬を規則正しく服用します。

Watashi wa kono okusuri o itsumo nondemasu.

3. Please call a doctor.

お医者さんを呼んで下さい。

Oisha o yonde kudasai.

4. Please call an ambulance.

救急車を呼んで下さい。

Kyūkyūsha o yonde kudasai.

5. It hurts here.

ここが痛いです。

Koko ga itai desu.

RUSSIAN
1. Please give me something for
Дайте пожалуйста, средство от
Daitye, pazhálusta, sredstvo ot

  a. a cold
простуды
prostōōdy

  b. a cough
кашля
káshlia

   c. constipation
     запора
     zapóra

   d. diarrhea
     расстройства желудка
     rasstróistva zhelúdka

   e. the flu
     гриппа
     gríppa

   f. headache
     головной боли
     golovnói bóli

   g. insect bites
     истребления насекомых
     ukōōsa nasekómykh

2. I take this medicine regularly.
   Я регулярно принимаю это лекарство
   Ya regulyārno prinimáyoo éto lekárstvo.

3. Please call me a doctor.
   Позовите, пожалуйста, врача.
   Pazaveétye, pozhálusta, vrachá.

4. Please call me an ambulance.
   Позовите, пожалуйста, скорую помощь.
   Pazaveétye, pozhálusta, skórooyoo pómoshch.

5. I have a pain here.
   Здесь болит
   Zdés boleēt.

HEBREW

1. I'd like something for . . . a cold / a cough / constipation / diarrhea / flu / headache / insect bites.

אֲנִי רוֹצֶה [רוֹצָה] מַשֶׁהוּ בִּשְׁבִיל צָנָה / שֵׁעוּל / עֲצִירוּת / שִׁלְשׁוּל / שַׁפַּעַת / כְּאֵב רֹאשׁ / עֲקִצַת חֶרֶק

(ah-nee ro-tzeh [ro-tzah] ma-she-hu bih-shveel . . . tzee-nah / shay-ul / ah-tzee rut / shil-shul / shah-pa-at / ki-ayv rosh / ah keetzat che-rek)

2. I take this medicine regularly.

אֲנִי לוֹקֵחַ [לוֹקַחַת] הַתְּרוּפָה הַזֹּאת בִּקְבִיעוּת

(ah-nee lo-kay-ach [lo-kah-chat] hah-tru-fah hah-zot bih-kvee-ut)

3. Get me a doctor please.

הַשֵּׂיג [הַשִּׂיגִי] לִי רוֹפֵא, בְּבַקָשָׁה

(ha-seeg [ha-see-gee] lee ro-feh bih-va-ka-shah)

4. Call an ambulance.

קְרָא [קְרְאִי] לְאַמְבּוּלַנְס

(ki-rah [ki-ree] li-am-bu-lantz)

5. I have a pain here.

יֵשׁ לִי כְּאֵב פֹּה

(yesh lee-ki-ayv poh)

13 | Home Again, but Not Home Free

You've just returned to the States, and everything is intact: your luggage, your camera equipment, your overseas business account . . . and your health. The trip was a total success. Now you can relax, right?

Not necessarily.

It's not quite time to let down your guard. First of all, travelers who have been away for more than a few days will need to adjust to returning home, just as they adjusted to leaving. For instance, you can expect to feel jet lag for the first few days back. Following the anti-jet lag instructions in chapter 1 will help ease the symptoms, but you should allow yourself at least one day per time zone crossed before you expect to feel like yourself again.

If you required any medical attention while you were away—for instance, if you had a broken bone set, or received any medication— it's important to let health care professionals in the States check you out and make sure you received competent care. Bring all medical records home with you, and check with your own physician or a specialist as soon as possible to make sure you were cared for properly.

Remember, it isn't quite time to congratulate yourself for returning home healthy. The verdict is still out. Many illnesses have a long incubation time, meaning that even though you acquired the disease while you were away, you won't feel the symptoms for days, weeks, or even months. For instance, a case of infectious hepatitis may take over a month to appear; a case of malaria, as much as several years (although usually just one to two weeks). If you become ill in the months following a trip abroad, it's important that you remind your physician of your trip, since it may play an important part in diagnosing what's wrong with you.

Be suspicious of flu-like symptoms (especially if nobody else you know has them, too, since the flu usually affects many people in a community), and of fever, jaundice, swollen glands, skin rash, or persistent diarrhea.

The diarrhea you came home with could be nothing but what it seems, or it could be any of a number of conditions. A sampling:

AMEBIASIS: A parasitic intestinal disease present throughout the world, it is commonly contracted by travelers through contaminated food or water, especially leafy vegetables that have not been properly washed before eating. Treatment includes fluid and electrolyte (salt, sugar, potassium, etc.) replacement plus medication (often the drug metronidazole, brand name Flagyl).

CHOLERA: Another intestinal disease caused by a microorganism, and transmitted to humans through contaminated water or food. Mostly found in Asia or Africa, the incubation time is just one to three days. The cholera vaccine is considered only 50 percent effective, so even protected travelers may contract the disease. Treatment consists of prompt replacement of fluids and electrolytes, and tetracycline antibiotics.

GIARDIASIS: Again, an intestinal infection, this time from a protozoan. Transmitted through contaminated drinking water. The diarrhea and other symptoms (abdominal discomfort, cramps, gas) usually occur one to three weeks after exposure. Treated with drugs, including Flagyl.

SHIGELLOSIS (bacillary dysentery): An acute infection of the intestinal tract, transmitted through contaminated food or water. The incubation period is just one to four days. Shigellosis is found worldwide, mostly in developing countries. Treated with fluid replacement, and antibiotic and antispasmodic medications.

THREADWORM (strongyloidiasis): A parasitic worm, common in the tropics, that lives in the intestines, and causes abdominal pain and tenderness, and often vomiting and diarrhea. Treated with drugs, including thiabendazole (Mintezol).

Many other illnesses can be mistaken for the flu, since symptoms can include fever, sweats, weakness, general aches and pains, headaches, and lethargy. Some of these threats to travelers:

BRUCELLOSIS: Caused by a microorganism usually transmitted to humans via contaminated milk and dairy products, or contact with animals. Brucellosis is most often reported from Latin American and

Mediterranean countries. The incubation time is one to three weeks, although sometimes months go by between infection and symptoms. Easy to misdiagnose because it mimics so many diseases (with symptoms of fatigue, headache, joint pain, loss of appetite, fever, chills, sweating), it is treated with antibiotics.

DENGUE FEVER (also called breakbone fever): This is a disease of the tropics and subtropics (Asia, the Pacific, Africa, the Caribbean, Central and South America). It is transmitted to humans by mosquitoes. The disease can be so mild as to go unnoticed, or symptoms can include high fever, chills, profuse nasal discharge, sore throat, severe headache, backache, joint and muscle pain, rash, insomnia, loss of appetite, weakness. Generally, the disease has an incubation time of three to sixteen days. The symptoms last for two or three days, then disappear, then recur. Dengue fever is seldom fatal (less than 3 percent of victims die), and treatment—which should be under a physician's direction—consists of pain relievers, fluids, and bedrest.

INFECTIOUS HEPATITIS: A viral disease of the liver, hepatitis is transmitted mainly through contaminated food and water. It is a risk to travelers in underdeveloped parts of Latin America, the Middle East, Asia, and Africa. The incubation period is two to six weeks, and the initial symptoms, which resemble flu, include weakness, muscle aches, headaches, fever, loss of appetite, nausea, and vomiting. The urine may turn dark, and stools may become lighter and yellowish. Then, after four to seven days, symptoms may become more severe, including diarrhea, itching, more severe nausea and vomiting, and usually jaundice (a yellowish tinge to the skin and the whites of the eyes). There is no specific treatment, but most people recover on their own, with bedrest, within six weeks.

LASSA FEVER: An African virus probably transmitted through contaminated food, or from humans with the disease. Incubation period ranges from one to twenty-four days, with the average being two weeks. The disease is often mild, characterized by a fever. Again, the nature of the symptoms makes it difficult to diagnose, and easy to mistake for the flu: fever, chills, headache, malaise, muscle pain. There may also be loss of appetite, vomiting, and chest pain. The symptoms last from one week to a month. Mild cases are treated with aspirin; more severe cases may require the experimental drug ribavirin.

MALARIA: Malaria prophylaxis is not foolproof, so travelers who have taken precautions against the disease as well as unprotected travelers may still come down with a case. A mosquito-borne disease, malaria usually has an incubation period of one to two weeks, but depending on the type of malaria, symptoms can appear months, or even years, after a trip to the tropics. The symptoms of malaria are also flu-like: general malaise, headache, body aches, fever, chills. Once diagnosed, malaria is usually quickly and completely cured with medication, including chloroquine (Aralen), hydroxychloroquine (Plaquenil), sulfadoxine and pyrimethamine (Fansidar), and others.

TYPHOID FEVER: Caused by a *Salmonella* organism, and passed to people from contaminated food (especially undercooked meats and shellfish), water, milk, and dairy products. Typhoid fever is primarily a disease of developing countries in Africa, Asia, and Central and South America. The incubation period is usually about ten days, but can range from three days to two months. Symptoms include headache, lethargy, fever, chills, cough, abdominal discomfort, rash, and sometimes constipation or diarrhea. The vaccine is not foolproof. Typhoid fever is usually treated with the antibiotics ampicillin or chloramphenicol.

TRYPANOSOMIASIS (African sleeping sickness): A disease carried by the African tsetse fly. The incubation time is ten days or longer (some forms of the disease can occur six months to several years after infection), and the main symptoms are fever, weakness, fatigue, rapid heartbeat. If not diagnosed and treated, African sleeping sickness is usually fatal. But with medical therapy, most patients survive. The disease is treated with the drugs suramin and pentamidine, available from the Centers for Disease Control.

YELLOW FEVER: A virus transmitted by mosquitoes, yellow fever is found in the tropics, especially central Africa and South America. The incubation time is three to six days. In mild cases, the only symptoms may be fever and headache. The disease resembles the flu except that there is no nasal discharge. In more severe cases, the symptoms include jaundice and internal bleeding. Yellow fever is rare in travelers, most of whom receive vaccinations before visiting areas where the disease is prevalent.

Other diseases that travelers to developing countries may bring back with them:

CHAGAS' DISEASE (also called American Trypanosomiasis): An illness endemic in rural parts of Central and South America, the parasite that causes Chagas' disease usually enters the human body through the bite of a large insect called the reduviid bug. Also called the vinchuca, the barbeiro, or the kissing or assassin bug, the insect that transmits Chagas' disease is almost an inch long, with a smooth, oval, brownish-colored body. The bug's bite is usually on the face. About a week after the bite, a hard, violet-hued swelling appears on the spot where the parasite entered the body—an important clue to diagnosis. The parasites travel through the bloodstream and invade the heart, brain, liver, and spleen. Untreated, about 10 percent of Chagas' victims will die within the first three months from acute heart infection. The remaining 90 percent, however, will appear to recover completely. The parasites, however, remain latent in the body, and can surface after ten or twenty years in the form of chronic heart disease.

Chagas' disease is rare in travelers, and is primarily a risk to hikers and campers in rural Central and South America. The only way to prevent Chagas' disease is to prevent the insect bites that introduce the parasites. Check all sleeping quarters carefully for insects, use insecticides on all exposed parts of the body, those containing N,N-diethyl-meta-toluamide—DEET—are best, and use a bed net if sleeping in a rural area of Central or South America. Vaccines for Chagas' disease are still in the experimental stage.

Chagas' disease can be detected by a blood test. It can be treated in its early stage by the drug benznidazol (Ragonil), which is available in South America, or by the medication nifurtimox (Lampit), which is available through the CDC. Once the disease is chronic, however, there is no treatment.

ENCEPHALITIS: Viral encephalitis is an infection and inflammation of the brain cells, caused by a virus that is passed to people primarily from mosquitoes. The disease occurs worldwide. There is a three- to ten-day incubation period. Symptoms include fever, headache, stiff neck, sore throat, nausea, and vomiting, which may progress to drowsiness and confusion, stupor, coma, and convulsions. People with mild cases of encephalitis recover completely, while those with more severe attacks (which are rare, but most often found in the very old or very young) may suffer permanent neurological damage, or death. There is no specific treatment (except for a specific type of encephalitis caused by the herpes simplex type I virus). Doctors try to ease the symptoms, keep the patient comfortable and well-nourished, and allow the body's immune system to fight the infection. (There is a vaccine to prevent Japanese B encephalitis, found in much of Asia, but the only way to protect most travelers against encephalitis is to prevent insect bites.)

FILARIASIS: A parasitic disease of the tropics transmitted to humans by mosquitoes and black flies. The disease has an incubation period of eight to twelve months (although sometimes as little as two or three). Symptoms include fever, headache, chills, cough, sweats, nausea, vomiting, and muscle pain. Sometimes, symptoms include a tender spot on the legs and abdomen, which spreads, or extreme swelling of the arms, legs, breasts, or genitalia. Other forms of filariasis—river blindness and Loa loa—affect the skin, causing either nodules under the skin, an itching rash, lesions on the eyes, or areas of allergic inflammation. All forms are treated with drugs, including antibiotics, antihistamines, and specific medications to kill the parasites. In severe cases with limb swelling, surgery may be necessary.

HEMORRHAGIC FEVERS: A diverse group of illnesses resulting from viruses (usually transmitted by ticks, mosquitoes, or animals), hemorrhagic fevers are linked by their symptoms: high fever, and bleeding from the nose, gastrointestinal tract, and genitourinary tract. Hemorrhagic fevers are present in Africa, South America, U.S.S.R., and India. Untreated, they can lead to shock and finally death. There is no specific treatment, but doctors can treat individual symptoms.

LEISHMANIASIS: Another parasite, transmitted to humans by sandfly bites in the tropics. Incubation is three weeks to eighteen months (two months average). Symptoms can include fever, rapid heartbeat, diarrhea, cough, skin lesions. Treated with a variety of drugs, most of which must be administered in a hospital by injection.

MENINGOCOCCAL MENINGITIS: An infection and inflammation of the membranes covering the brain and spinal cord—the meninges. Caused by a bacterium, the disease usually occurs in epidemics. The incubation time is one day to three weeks. Symptoms include skin rash, fever, chills, headache, convulsions, nausea, vomiting, confusion, delirium, stiff neck and back. The disease can end in permanent disability (blindness, deafness, mental impairment) unless quickly diagnosed and treated. If diagnosed early enough, however, doctors can successfully treat most cases. Meningococcal meningitis is treated with antibiotics such as penicillin and chloramphenicol, among others.

PLAGUE: A rodent disease passed to humans through flea bites, plague occurs worldwide, primarily in the southwestern United States, southeast Asia, and South America. The incubation time is from one to twelve days, and the symptoms include fever, extreme exhaustion, muscular pains, enlarged lymph nodes, chills, rapid heartbeat, headache, vomiting, and delirium. Plague is usually fatal if undiagnosed and untreated, but can be cured with prompt and proper drug therapy, usually the antibiotics streptomycin, chloramphenicol (Chloromycetin), tetracycline, or gentamicin (Garamycin).

SCHISTOSOMIASIS (Bilharziasis): A parasite acquired from contaminated fresh water used for washing, bathing, swimming, or drinking. Present in Africa, South America, Asia, and the Caribbean. The first sign is a skin rash and itching, followed by headache, muscle aches, abdominal pain, and diarrhea. Symptoms often disappear and recur, and one to two months later the victim may suffer from a high fever, cough, pains in the joints, hives, diarrhea. Treated with drugs, including praziquantel (Biltricide).

One other post-voyage disease risk to travelers comes from souvenirs. For instance, eating or drinking out of poorly glazed pottery—a popular souvenir from Mexico and other Latin American countries— can cause lead poisoning over time. And contaminated animal skins, furs, or yarns can transmit diseases such as anthrax.

Most travelers' diseases run their course in people who are otherwise healthy, and then disappear. Or, diagnosed promptly, they can be quickly and easily cured. These diseases can be more of a risk for the very old, the very young, pregnant women, and people who are ill or on certain medications.

Actually, the risk to travelers of acquiring most of the conditions listed above is relatively small, because they are generally not present in facilities that cater to American tourists. Proper food and water (drinking and swimming) precautions, and protection against insect bites, reduce the risk to almost zero.

If you or your physician suspect a tropical illness, or if you began treatment for an exotic disease while you were away, you might be best cared for by a physician who specializes in treating these disorders. Medical specialties that encompass travelers' health are emporiatrics (from the Greek word for traveler), tropical medicine (dealing specifically with diseases common to warm climates), and infectious diseases. Many cities, hospitals, universities, and medical schools now have travelers' health clinics specifically to educate travelers about proper precautions, and to handle diseases and medical conditions not commonly seen in the States.

These clinics are excellent sources of pre-trip information as well as post-trip care. Most provide physical examinations, which include any necessary immunizations. They also offer advice on the food and water safety, and special health concerns—such as tropical diseases, stinging insects, or extreme heat, cold, or altitude—for any destination. Some even provide their patients with a phone number to call in case of emergency abroad: Clinic doctors can either recommend a physician overseas, or speak to a foreign physician for you, should the need arise, to ensure you are receiving proper care.

Travelers who have spent more than a week or two in rural areas of an undeveloped country may choose to visit a travelers' clinic for a post-trip exam, which will probably include a complete blood count, liver function tests, stool examination to test for parasites, and tests for such nonparasitic infections as brucellosis, shigellosis, and Salmonella infection.

To find a travelers' health clinic near you, call local hospitals and universities; most have public relations or community relations departments that can answer your questions, or you can ask to be connected with the infectious disease department. You can also call the local public health department for information. The following is a partial listing of travelers' health clinics across the country:

CALIFORNIA
Travelers' Clinic
University of California, San Diego, Medical Center
(619) 543-5787

Tropical Medicine Clinic
Department of Epidemiology and International Health
University of California, San Francisco
(415) 476-4937

CONNECTICUT
The Center for International Health
Mansfield Professional Park
Storrs
(203) 487-0002

The Tropical Medicine and International Travelers Clinic
Yale–New Haven Medical Center
New Haven
(203) 785-2476

ILLINOIS
Travelers Immunization and Preparation Services (TIPS)
Holy Family Ambulatory Care Center
Wheeling
(312) 520-0100

LOUISIANA
The Ochsner Travelers' Clinic
New Orleans
(504) 838-4005

MARYLAND
International Travel Clinic
The Johns Hopkins Medical Institutions
Baltimore
(301) 955-8931

MASSACHUSETTS
Traveler's Center
Tufts–New England Medical Center
Boston
(617) 956-0159

MICHIGAN
Travel Health
Henry Ford Hospital
Detroit
(313) 876-2561

NEW YORK
International Health Care Service
The New York Hospital–Cornell Medical Center
New York City
(212) 472-4284

Travel and Immunization Center
Long Island Jewish–Hillside Medical Center
New Hyde Park (Queens)
(718) 470-7290

Tropical Disease Center
Lenox Hill Hospital
New York City
(212) 439-2477

OHIO
Traveler's Clinic
University Hospitals of Cleveland
(216) 844-3295

PENNSYLVANIA
Traveler's Clinic
Milton S. Hershey Medical Center
Pennsylvania State University
Hershey
(717) 534-8161

TRAVELHEALTH Center
Medical College of Pennsylvania
Philadelphia
(215) 842-6465

VIRGINIA
Traveler's Clinic
University of Virginia
Charlottesville
(804) 924-9677

WASHINGTON
Travel—Tropical Medicine Clinic
University Hospital
University of Washington
Seattle
(206) 543-7902

WASHINGTON, D.C.
Traveler's Medical Service
(202) 466-8109

Travelers Clinic
The George Washington University Medical Center
(202) 676-8467
(also has clinics at Washington National Airport and Dulles International
Airport)

CANADA
Travel and Inoculation Service
Toronto General Hospital
(416) 595-3670

14 | Health Guide to the World

The world is a large and varied place, and so, too, are the health risks to the traveler in different corners of the globe. And since prevention is infinitely preferable to treatment, the following is a region-by-region guide to world health hazards.

The general information under each regional heading is adapted from the 1986 edition of the Centers for Disease Control's publication *Health Information for International Travel.* (The book is updated annually, in June.) The information on malaria risks is compiled from the same source (for information on malaria prevention see chapter 1). To obtain a copy of the CDC's book, contact the U.S. Government Printing Office in Washington, D.C. (202) 783-3238.

The country-by-country immunization recommendations, and the key to reading the symbols, are reprinted from the International Association for Medical Assistance to Travelers' (IAMAT) "World Immunization Chart." For more information on IAMAT, see chapter 1.

Remember, protection against disease includes not just inoculations and malaria prophylaxis when necessary, but also food, water, insect, and parasite precautions. For an almost certainly healthy vacation or business trip, follow the tips for insect prevention in chapter 1, and the food and water precautions in chapter 3. Also, be careful about swimming in fresh water without first ascertaining its safety, as in much of the world contaminated water can lead to schistosomiasis or other illness. And avoid walking barefoot, since soil in rural areas may contain parasites that can enter the body through the soles of the feet.

Finally, remember that disease conditions around the world are constantly changing, and the immunization requirements and other recommended health precautions change along with them. Use the following section as a guide to the health risks of your destination, but check with one of the information sources listed in chapter 1 at least a month before your trip to receive the most up-to-the-minute advice.

WORLD IMMUNIZATION CHART
as of October 15, 1985

Immunization Code

C = Cholera, D = Dengue Fever, H = Viral Hepatitis, Type A (Immune globulin), M = Meningococcal Meningitis, P = Plague, Ra = Rabies, T = epidemic louse borne Typhus, Td = Typhoid Fever, Y = Yellow Fever, R = Routine Immunizations (Diphtheria, Polio,* Tetanus). Vaccination not required for children: ∝ = under 3 months of age, β = under six months of age, γ = under 1 year of age, δ = under 13 months of age.

*Persons who have been immunized with polio vaccine and intend to travel to areas with increased risk (inadequate sanitation, current epidemics) should be given a booster dose of either trivalent oral polio vaccine (TOPV) or inactivated polio vaccine (IPV). Partially vaccinated and unvaccinated persons under 18 years should complete the vaccination series or be given the full series with TOPV.
Partially vaccinated and unvaccinated adults should receive only IPV.

① Vaccination certificate required on arrival from all countries.
② Vaccination certificate is required from travelers coming from infected areas.
③ Vaccination certificate is required from travelers coming from the following countries and areas, which are regarded as infected:

Africa: Angola, Benin, Botswana, Burundi, Cameroon, Central African Republic, Chad, Congo, Equatorial Guinea, Ethiopia, Gabon, Gambia, Ghana, Guinea, Guinea-Bissau, Ivory Coast, Kenya, Liberia, Malawi, Mali, Mauritania, Niger, Nigeria, Rwanda, São Tomé and Principe, Senegal, Sierra Leone, Somalia, Sudan (south of 15 N latitude), Tanzania, Togo, Uganda, Upper Volta, Zaire, Zambia.
Americas: Belize, Bolivia, Brazil, Colombia, Costa Rica, Ecuador, French Guiana, Guatemala, Guyana, Honduras, Nicaragua, Panama, Peru, Suriname, Trinidad, Venezuela.

④ Vaccination is recommended when traveling outside the usual areas visited by tourists, traveling extensively in the interior of the country, or on working assignments.
⑤ Vaccination is recommended for all travelers for their own protection.
⑥ Because of the moderate and short-lived protection given by cholera vaccine, the best prevention is to follow meticulous personal hygiene. IAMAT advises immunization only for people living and working in endemic areas under inadequate sanitary conditions, and for persons with impaired defense mechanisms (previous surgery for duodenal or gastric ulcer, antacid therapy, achlorhydria). Users of cannabis might be interested to know that smoking marijuana reduces the acid secretion of the stomach, making the user susceptible to cholera infection while traveling in endemic areas.
⑦ Travelers leaving the country are requested to possess a vaccination certificate if they are going to countries which still demand such certificates.
⑧ Travelers on scheduled airlines whose flights have originated outside the areas regarded as infected and who are in transit through these areas, are not required to possess a certificate provided they have remained at the scheduled airport or in the adjacent town during transit.
⑨ *Except:* Travelers arriving from a noninfected area and staying less than 2 weeks in the country.

10 Vaccination is recommended only for persons who may be occupationally exposed to wild rodents (anthropologists, geologists, medical personnel, missionaries, etc.). The standard vaccination course must be completed before entering the plague infested area. Tourists traveling temporarily in the interior of the country will be sufficiently protected against plague by taking broad-spectrum antibiotics or sulfa-diazine.

11 A certificate is also required from travelers coming from Afghanistan, Bahrain, Bangladesh, Burma, India, Iraq, Malawi, Malaysia, Pakistan, Philippines, Saudi Arabia, Singapore, Thailand, Vietnam, and also from passengers of aircraft having called at an airport situated in an infected area.

12 Yellow fever vaccination is recommended for all travelers. It is required for all travelers arriving in or destined for that part of the Zaire south of 10° S.

13 Persons on working assignments (including family members over one year of age) are advised to have pre-exposure rabies inoculations. Although these will provide adequate initial protection, a bite by a potentially rabid animal would still require the full series of inoculations. Children should be cautioned not to pet dogs, cats, and other mammals.

14 Vaccination is recommended only for persons who may be occupationally exposed to wild rodents in the interior of the following states: Arizona, California, Colorado, New Mexico, and Oregon (scientific investigators, anthropologists, archaeologists, geologists, etc.).

15 Risk exists for persons living or working in the interior of the country (anthropologists, archaeologists, geologists, medical personnel, missionaries, etc.). Freedom from louse infestation is the most effective protection against typhus. Apply residual insecticide powder to clothes and follow meticulous personal hygiene. Production of typhus vaccine, which is no longer available in Canada or the United States, is being discontinued throughout the world. In case of illness, treatment with tetracyclines will cure completely.

16 The requirement applies only to travelers arriving in or destined for the Azores and Madeira. No certificate is, however, required from transit passengers at Funchal, Porto Santo, and Santa Maria.

17 A certificate is required from travelers who have been in or passed through an infected yellow fever area within 6 days prior to arrival.

18 The requirement does not apply to travelers arriving in São Vincente, Sal, Maio, Boa Vista and Santiago.

19 Children under one year of age shall be subjected to isolation or surveyance if indicated.

20 Potential risk of dengue fever exists. The disease is endemo-epidemic in this country (i.e., the virus is present at all times and may give rise to major outbreaks).

Description of the disease and protective measures. Commonly called "breakbone" fever, the disease starts with a sharp rise in temperature, severe headache, and muscular and joint pain. A bright red rash may appear on the fourth day. This virus disease is transmitted by the bite of the infected female *Aëdes aegypti* mosquito, a domestic species that breeds in artificial water containers both outside and inside living quarters and bites during daylight. For protection apply anti-mosquito measures: Wear long-sleeved shirts and long trousers; apply mosquito repellents to the exposed parts of the skin. Dispose of such containers as bottles, jars, old tires; change water in flower vases or other standing containers frequently; ensure that window and door screens of living quarters fit tightly and are free of holes.

21   This country must be considered receptive to dengue fever. Intermittent epidemics in the past make renewed activity or reintroduction of the virus possible. For description of the disease and protective measures see also 20.

22   The disease is limited to the northern part of coastal Queensland.

23   Risk is limited to the coastal areas of the following states: Amapá, Pará, Maranháo, Piauí.

24   Risk is limited to the southern provinces of Yunnan, Guangxi, and Guangdong.

25   A cholera vaccination certificate is required from travelers intending to enter the Islands of Zanzibar and Pemba.

26   A yellow fever vaccination certificate is required from all travelers going to the provinces of Bocas del Toro and Darién.

27   Vaccination is advised for persons traveling extensively or on working assignments in the meningitis belt of Africa's northern savanna which stretches from the Red Sea to the Atlantic. Included are the following areas: Sudan: the southern two thirds; Chad: the southern half; Niger: the southern third; Burkina Faso: the entire country; Mali: the southern half; Mauritania: the southern third; Central African Republic: the northern third; Cameroon: the northern third; Nigeria: the northern half; Benin: the entire country; Togo: the northern third; Ghana: the border areas with Burkina Faso; Senegal: the northern third. Peak season: March–April.

The information on vaccination requirements has been compiled from data gathered by the World Health organization. IAMAT acknowledges the contribution of Dr. Scott B. Halstead on the geographical distribution of dengue fever.

AFRICA

In NORTHERN AFRICA—which includes the countries of Algeria, Egypt, Libya, Morocco, and Tunisia—the biggest risks to the traveler are food- and water-borne diseases such as dysentery and other diarrheal illness. Typhoid fever and viral hepatitis (type A) are common in some areas. Schistosomiasis (bilharziasis) is prevalent around the Nile River in Egypt, and in other countries in this region, too. Helminthic (parasitic worm) infections, brucellosis, and giardiasis are also common. Other hazards in this area include polio, trachoma (an eye infection), rabies, scorpion stings, and snake bites. The following diseases are also present, but are not considered to be a great risk for travelers: dengue fever, filariasis (in the Nile delta), leishmaniasis, malaria, relapsing fever, Rift Valley fever (a viral disease transmitted by mosquitoes or infected livestock), sandfly fever, typhus, plague (in parts of Libya).

In SOUTHERN AFRICA—which includes the countries of Botswana, Lesotho, Namibia, St. Helena, South Africa, and Swaziland—such diseases as malaria, plague, relapsing fever, Rift Valley fever, tick bite fever, and typhus have been reported. Except for malaria, however, they are not considered to be major risks to travelers. Trypanosomiasis (sleeping sickness) is a hazard in Botswana and Namibia, and in the northern Transvaal in South Africa. Food- and water-borne diseases, particularly amebiasis and typhoid fever, are common in some areas. Schistosomiasis (bilharziasis) is common in the northern and eastern parts of South Africa. Snake bites may also be a hazard.

In SUB-SAHARAN AFRICA—which includes the over three-dozen countries which complete the African continent—disease risks are high, since the region lies entirely within the tropics. Malaria occurs throughout the area (with the exception of several of the islands off Africa's coast, and altitudes over ten thousand feet. Filariasis, leishmaniasis, and trypanosomiasis (sleeping sickness) are present, as are relapsing fever, and typhus transmitted by lice, fleas, or ticks. Plague has been reported from Kenya, Madagascar, Mozambique, the United Republic of Tanzania, and Zaire. Tungiasis, a flea-borne disease, is widespread in western Africa. Scattered cases of yellow fever are reported, with an occasional outbreak that is more extensive.

Food- and water-borne diseases are a great risk in this area. These include schistosomiasis (bilharziasis), parasitic worm infections, dysentery and diarrheal illness, giardiasis, typhoid fever, and viral hepatitis. Polio is endemic in most of these countries except Mauritius, Réunion, and the Seychelles. Trachoma (an eye infection) is widespread. Hemorrhagic fevers and Lassa fever are also a risk. Epidemics of meningococcal meningitis may occur throughout tropical Africa, especially in the savanna areas during the dry season. Other hazards include rabies and snake bites.

ALGERIA
Immunization: Y2γ, H4, Td4, R5
Malaria risk: Very limited risk in Sahara region.

ANGOLA
Immunization: C2, Y1γ, H5, Td5, R5, D21
Malaria risk: Throughout country.
 Chloroquine resistance.

BENIN
Immunization: Y1γ, H5, M27, Td5, R5, D21
Malaria risk: Throughout country.

BOTSWANA
Immunization: H5, T15, Td5, R5
Malaria risk: In northern part of country.

BURKINA FASO (formerly Upper Volta)
Immunization: Y1γ, H5, M27, Ra13, R5
Malaria risk: Throughout country.

BURUNDI
Immunization: C6, Y2γ,5, H5, T15, Td5, R5

Malaria risk: Throughout country.
 Chloroquine resistance.

CAMEROON
Immunization: C6, Y1γ, H5, M27, T15, Td5, R5, D21
Malaria risk: Throughout country.
 Chloroquine resistance.

CAPE VERDE
Immunization: C2, Y2γ,18,5, H5, Td5, R5
Malaria risk: None.

CENTRAL AFRICAN REPUBLIC
Immunization: Y1γ, H5, M27, Ra13, Td5, R5
Malaria risk: Throughout country.
 Chloroquine resistance.

CHAD
Immunization: C6, Y5γ, M27, H5, Ra13, T15, Td5, R5
Malaria risk: Throughout country.

COMORO ISLANDS
Immunization: H5, Td5, R5
Malaria risk: Throughout country.
 Chloroquine resistance.

CONGO
Immunization: C6, Y1γ,9,5, H5, T15, Td5, R5, D21
Malaria risk: Throughout country. Chloroquine resistance.

DJIBOUTI
Immunization: Y2γ, H4, Td4, R5, D21
Malaria risk: Throughout country.

EGYPT
Immunization: Y2,3γ, H5, Ra13, Td5, R5
Malaria risk: In rural areas of Nile delta, El Faiyum area, the oases, and part of southern (upper) Egypt.

EQUATORIAL GUINEA
Immunization: Y2,5, H5, Td5, R5, D21
Malaria risk: Throughout country.

ETHIOPIA
Immunization: Y2γ,5, Ra13, T15, Td4, R5, D21
Malaria risk: Throughout country, except not in Addis Ababa and above 6,500 feet (two thousand meters).

GABON
Immunization: Y2γ,5, H5, Td5, R5, D21
Malaria risk: Throughout country. Chloroquine resistance.

GAMBIA
Immunization: Y1γ, H5, Td5, R5, D21
Malaria risk: Throughout country.

GHANA
Immunization: C6, Y2γ,3,5, H5, M27, Td5, R5, D21
Malaria risk: Throughout country.

GUINEA
Immunization: Y2γ,5, H5, Ra13, Td5, R5, D21
Malaria risk: Throughout country.

GUINEA-BISSAU
Immunization: Y2,3γ,5, H5, Ra13, Td5, R5, D21
Malaria risk: Throughout country.

IVORY COAST
Immunization: Y1γ, H5, TD5, R5, D21
Malaria risk: Throughout country.

KENYA
Immunization: Y2,3γ,5, H4, Td4, R5
Malaria risk: Throughout country, including game parks, but not in Nairobi or over 8,000 feet (2,500 meters). Chloroquine resistance.

LESOTHO
Immunization: C2, Y2, H4, P10, Td4, R5
Malaria risk: None.

LIBERIA
Immunization: C6, Y2,3γ,5, H5, Td5, R5, D21
Malaria risk: Throughout country.

LIBYAN ARAB JAMAHIRIYA (Libya)
Immunization: Y2γ, H4, Td4, R5
Malaria risk: Very limited risk in southwest part of country.

MADAGASCAR
Immunization: C2, Y2,3, H5, P10, Td5, R5
Malaria risk: In coastal areas. Limited risk in Antananarivo, Andramasina, Antsirabe and Manjakandriana. Chloroquine resistance.

MALAWI
Immunization: Y2,5, H5, Td5, R5
Malaria risk: Throughout country. Chloroquine resistance.

MALI
Immunization: C2, Y1,9,5, H5, M27, Td5, R5
Malaria risk: Throughout country.

MAURITANIA
Immunization: Y1γ,9, H5, M27, Ra13, Td5, R5
Malaria risk: Throughout country, except not in the northern areas: Dakhlet-Nouadhibou, Inchiri, Adrar, and Tiris-Zemour.

MAURITIUS
Immunization: Y2,3γ, R5
Malaria risk: In rural areas, except not on Rodrigues Island.

MOROCCO
Immunization: H4, Ra13, Td4, R5
Malaria risk: Very limited risk in rural areas of coastal provinces.

MOZAMBIQUE
Immunization: C1, Y2γ, H5, P10, Ra13, Td5, R5
Malaria risk: Throughout country. Chloroquine resistance.

NAMIBIA
Immunization: Y2,3,8, H4, P10, Td4, R5
Malaria risk: In all areas of Ovamboland and Caprivi Strip. Chloroquine resistance.

NIGER
Immunization: Y1γ, H5, M27, T15, Td5, R5
Malaria risk: Throughout country.

NIGERIA
Immunization: C6,7, Y1γ, H5, M27, Ra13, T15, Td5, R5, D21
Malaria risk: Throughout country.

RÉUNION (France)
Immunization: Y2γ, R5
Malaria risk: None.

RWANDA
Immunization: C6, Y1γ, H5, T15, Td5, R5
Malaria risk: Throughout country. Chloroquine resistance.

ST. HELENA (U.K.)
Immunization: R5
Malaria risk: None.

SÃO TOMÉ AND PRÍNCIPE
Immunization: Y1γ,9,5, H5, Td5, R5
Malaria risk: Throughout country.

SENEGAL
Immunization: Y1, H5, M27, Td5, R5
Malaria risk: Throughout country.

SEYCHELLES
Immunization: R5, D21
Malaria risk: None.

SIERRA LEONE
Immunization: Y2,5, H5, Ra13, Td5, R5, D21
Malaria risk: Throughout country.

SOMALIA
Immunization: C2, Y2,5, H5, Td5, R5, D21
Malaria risk: Throughout country.

SOUTH AFRICA
Immunization: Y2,3,8, H4, P10, T15, Td4, R5
Malaria risk: In rural areas (including game parks) in the north, east, and western low altitude areas of Transvaal and Natal coast. Isolated reports of chloroquine resistance.

SUDAN
Immunization: C2,6, Y2,3,5, H5, M27, P10, Ra13, Td5, R5
Malaria risk: Throughout country. Chloroquine resistance in the northern provinces.

SWAZILAND
Immunization: Y2, H4, P10, Ra13, T15, Td4, R5
Malaria risk: In all lowland areas. Isolated reports of chloroquine resistance.

TOGO
Immunization: Y1, H5, M27, T15, Td5, R5, D21
Malaria risk: Throughout country.

TUNISIA
Immunization: Y2γ, H4, Td4, R5
Malaria risk: None.

UGANDA
Immunization: C6, Y1γ, H4, Ra13, Td4, R5
Malaria risk: Throughout country. Chloroquine resistance.

UNITED REPUBLIC OF TANZANIA
Immunization: C25, Y2,3γ,5, H5, P10, Ra13, Td5, R5
Malaria risk: Throughout country. Chloroquine resistance.

ZAIRE
Immunization: C6, Y2,12γ, H5, P10, T15, Td5, R5, D21
Malaria risk: Throughout country. Chloroquine resistance.

ZAMBIA
Immunization: Y2γ, H5, T15, Td5, R5
Malaria risk: Throughout country. Chloroquine resistance.

ZIMBABWE (formerly Rhodesia)
Immunization: Y2, H4, T15, Td4, R5
Malaria risk: Throughout country, except not in city of Harare. Chloroquine resistance.

NORTH AMERICA

In NORTH AMERICA—which includes the United States of America, Canada, Bermuda, Greenland, St. Pierre and Miquelon—the risk of disease is extremely low, and certainly no greater than what a traveler would face at home, no matter where that is. One of the greatest health risks is from the extremely low temperatures in the winter, especially if a traveler is unaccustomed to cold climates. In terms of disease, there are isolated cases of plague, rabies (in wildlife and bats), Rocky Mountain spotted fever, tularemia (also called rabbit fever, a disease with flu-like symptoms transmitted by an animal bite or scratch), and encephalitis. Poisonous snakes, poison ivy, and poison oak may be a hazard.

UNITED STATES OF AMERICA
Immunization: R5, P14
Malaria risk: None.

CANADA
Immunization: R5
Malaria risk: None.

BERMUDA
Immunization: R5
Malaria risk: None.

GREENLAND (Denmark)
Immunization: R5
Malaria risk: None.

ST. PIERRE AND MIQUELON
Immunization: R5
Malaria risk: None.

CENTRAL AMERICA

CENTRAL AMERICA includes the countries of Belize, Costa Rica, El Salvador, Guatemala, Honduras, Mexico, Nicaragua, and Panama. Diseases that are found in all of these countries include malaria, leishmaniasis, and Chagas' disease (American trypanosomiasis). Polio is reported from all countries except Costa Rica and Panama. Rabies (usually spread by dogs and bats) is widespread. Dengue fever and certain types of encephalitis may also occur. There have been cases of onchocerciasis (river blindness) in parts of Mexico and Guatemala.

Food- and water-borne diseases include typhoid fever, amebic and bacillary dysentery and other diarrheal diseases. Viral hepatitis occurs throughout this region, and parasitic worm infections are common. Brucellosis occurs in the northern part of Central America, and paragonimiasis (Oriental lung fluke, a parasitic disease) has been reported in Costa Rica and Panama. Snakes may be a hazard.

BELIZE (formerly British Honduras)
Immunization: Y2, H4, Td4, R5, D21
Malaria risk: In rural areas, except no risk in Belize District.

COSTA RICA
Immunization: H4, Td4, R5, D21
Malaria risk: Limited risk in rural areas of Alajuela, Guanacaste, Limon, and Puntarenas provinces.

EL SALVADOR
Immunization: Y2β, H4, Td4, R5, D21
Malaria risk: In rural areas.

GUATEMALA
Immunization: Y2γ, H4, T15, Td4, R5, D21
Malaria risk: In rural areas, except not in central highlands.

HONDURAS
Immunization: Y2, H4, Td4, R5, D21
Malaria risk: In rural areas.

MEXICO
Immunization: Y2β, H4, Td4, R5, D21
Malaria risk: In rural areas, plus limited risk in major resorts on Pacific and Gulf coasts.

NICARAGUA
Immunization: H4, Td4, R5, D21
Malaria risk: In rural areas, plus risk exists on outskirts of following towns: Chinandega, Leon, Granada, Managua, Nandaime, and Tipitapa.

PANAMA
Immunization: Y26,4, H4, Td4, R5, D21
Malaria risk: In rural areas of Darien Province and Territories of Chiman and Puerto de Obaldia. Chloroquine resistance east of Canal Zone.

SOUTH AMERICA

TEMPERATE SOUTH AMERICA includes the countries of Argentina, Chile, the Falkland Islands (Malvinas), and Uruguay.

In Argentina, Chagas' disease (American trypanosomiasis) is widespread in rural areas, and outbreaks of malaria occur in the northwest. Leishmaniasis is reported from the northeastern part of Argentina. Hemorrhagic fever is endemic in part of the pampas, and in the center of the country. Food- and water-borne diseases, especially diarrhea caused by Salmonella, are relatively common in Argentina, but typhoid fever is not. Intestinal parasites are common in the coastal region of Argentina.

Viral hepatitis is widespread in Argentina, and reported from the other countries in this region as well. Tapeworms and typhoid fever are also reported from the other countries. Diseases such as rabies and anthrax, which are transmitted by animals, are present.

TROPICAL SOUTH AMERICA includes the countries of Bolivia, Brazil, Colombia, Ecuador, French Guiana, Guyana, Paraguay, Peru, Suriname, and Venezuela. Because of the tropical climate, there is a greater risk of disease in this region. Malaria, Chagas' disease (American trypanosomiasis), and leishmaniasis are found in all ten of these countries. Polio is also present in all areas, although it is uncommon in French Guiana, Guyana, and Suriname. Rabies has been reported from many of these countries. Onchocerciasis (river blindness) occurs in rural areas of Colombia, Ecuador, Venezuela, and northern Brazil. Meningococcal meningitis occurs in epidemic outbreaks in Brazil. Filariasis is endemic in parts of Brazil, French Guiana, Guyana, Suriname, and possibly, Venezuela. Plague has been reported from Bolivia, Brazil, Ecuador, and Peru. Yellow fever is a risk in forest areas of all these countries except Paraguay and areas east of the Andes. Epidemics of viral encephalitis and dengue fever occur in the northern part of this region. Bartonellosis (Oroya fever), a sandfly-borne disease, occurs in parts of the Andes. Typhus, borne by lice, is common in mountain areas of Colombia and Peru.

Food- and water-borne diseases are common in this region, and include amebiasis, diarrheal diseases, parasitic worm infections, and viral hepatitis. Schistosomiasis (bilharziasis) is found in Brazil, Suriname, and parts of Venezuela. Paragonimiasis (Oriental lung fluke, a parasitic disease) has been reported from Ecuador and Peru. Brucellosis is common. A viral hemorrhagic fever that may be food-borne has been reported from Bolivia. Snakes and leeches may be a hazard in some areas.

ARGENTINA
Immunization: H4, Td4, R5
Malaria risk: In rural areas near Bolivian
 border.

BOLIVIA
Immunization: Y2,3,5, H4, P10, T15,
 Td4, R5
Malaria risk: In most rural areas. Chloroquine resistance.

BRAZIL
Immunization: Y2β,4, H4, P10, Td4, R5, D21,23
Malaria risk: In most rural areas, plus in urban areas of interior Amazon River basin. Chloroquine resistance.

CHILE
Immunization: H4, Td4, R5
Malaria risk: None.

COLOMBIA
Immunization: Y4, H4, Td4, R5, D20
Malaria risk: In rural areas, except no risk in Bogotá and vicinity. Chloroquine resistance.

ECUADOR
Immunization: Y4, H4, P10, T15, Td4, R5
Malaria risk: In many areas of country. Chloroquine resistance.

FALKLAND ISLANDS (MALVINAS) (U.K.)
Immunization: R5
Malaria risk: None

FRENCH GUIANA
Immunization: Y1γ,9,5, H4, Td4, R5, D20
Malaria risk: Throughout country. Chloroquine resistance.

GUYANA
Immunization: Y2,3,5, H4, Td4, R5, D20
Malaria risk: In rural areas in Rupununi and northwest regions. Chloroquine resistance.

PARAGUAY
Immunization: Y2β, H4, Td4, R5
Malaria risk: In rural areas bordering Brazil.

PERU
Immunization: Y2β,4, H4, P10, T15, Td4, R5
Malaria risk: In rural areas, except no risk in Lima and vicinity and coastal area south of Lima. Chloroquine resistance in northern provinces bordering Brazil.

SURINAME
Immunization: Y2,4, H4, Td4, R5, D20
Malaria risk: In rural areas, except no risk in Paramaribo District and northern coastal areas. Chloroquine resistance.

URUGUAY
Immunization: R5
Malaria risk: None.

VENEZUELA
Immunization: Y4, H4, P10, Td4, R5, D20
Malaria risk: In rural areas of Apure, Bolivar, Barinas, Merida, Tachira, and Zulia States. Chloroquine resistance.

THE CARIBBEAN ISLANDS

Malaria has been eradicated in much of this region, with the exception of Haiti and the western part of the Dominican Republic. Polio is also endemic in the Dominican Republic and Haiti. Leishmaniasis is present in the Dominican Republic, and tularemia (a flu-like illness transmitted by the bite or scratch of small animals, often rabbits) has been found in Haiti. Yellow fever is a risk in Trinidad and Tobago. Filariasis and dengue fever are present throughout the area. Food- and water-borne diseases such as bacillary and amebic dysenteries are common. Viral hepatitis is a risk in the more northern islands. Schistosomiasis is a risk in all the islands, but especially in the Dominican Republic, Guadeloupe, Martinique, Puerto Rico, and Saint Lucia. Rabies (particularly transmitted by the mongoose) is present on several islands.

Other hazards include spiny sea urchins, coral, jellyfish, and snakes.

ANTIGUA AND BARBUDA
Immunization: Y2γ, R5, D20
Malaria risk: None.

BAHAMAS
Immunization: Y2γ, R5, D21
Malaria risk: None.

BARBADOS
Immunization: Y2,3γ, R5, D20
Malaria risk: None.

BRITISH VIRGIN ISLANDS
Immunization: R5, D20
Malaria risk: None.

CAYMAN ISLANDS (U.K.)
Immunization: R5, D21
Malaria risk: None.

CUBA
Immunization: H4, Td4, R5, D21
Malaria risk: None.

DOMINICA
Immunization: Y2γ, R5, D20
Malaria risk: None.

DOMINICAN REPUBLIC
Immunization: H4, Td4, R5, D20
Malaria risk: In rural areas, with highest risk in areas bordering Haiti.

GRENADA
Immunization: Y2, R5, D20
Malaria risk: None.

GUADELOUPE
Immunization: Y2γ, R5, D20
Malaria risk: None.

HAITI
Immunization: Y2, H5, Td5, R5, D20
Malaria risk: Throughout country.

JAMAICA
Immunization: Y2γ, R5, D20
Malaria risk: None.

MARTINIQUE (France)
Immunization: Y2γ, R5, D20
Malaria risk: None.

MONTSERRAT
Immunization: Y2γ, R5, D20
Malaria risk: None.

NETHERLANDS ANTILLES
Immunization: Y2β, R5, D20
Malaria risk: None.

PUERTO RICO
Immunization: R5, D20
Malaria risk: None.

ST. CHRISTOPHER (SAINT KITTS)
AND NEVIS (U.K.)
Immunization: Y2γ, R5, D20
Malaria risk: None.

SAINT LUCIA
Immunization: Y2,3γ, R5, D20
Malaria risk: None.

SAINT VINCENT AND THE
GRENADINES
Immunization: Y2γ, R5, D20
Malaria risk: None.

TRINIDAD AND TOBAGO
Immunization: Y2γ,4, R5, D20
Malaria risk: None.

U.S. VIRGIN ISLANDS
Immunization: R5, D20
Malaria risk: None.

ASIA

The vast Asian continent can be divided into four regions, and each region's health risks can be discussed separately.

EAST ASIA includes the countries of China (mainland China and Taiwan), the Democratic People's Republic of Korea (North Korea), Hong Kong, Japan, Macao, Mongolia, and the Republic of Korea (South Korea).

In this area, malaria occurs only in China, particularly in the southern provinces. Leishmaniasis, plague, trachoma (an infectious eye disease), brucellosis, and polio are also found in China. Filariasis, tick-borne encephalitis, and typhus are reported from China and the Republic of Korea. Typhus is also present in some river valleys of Japan. Epidemics of dengue fever, hemorrhagic fever, and Japanese encephalitis may occur in this area.

Food- and water-borne diseases such as diarrheal illness and viral hepatitis are common in most of these countries. Schistosomiasis (bilharziasis) is a risk around the waterways of southeastern and eastern China. Parasitic diseases such as clonorchiasis (Oriental liver fluke) and paragonimiasis (Oriental lung fluke) are present in China, Japan, and the Republic of Korea; fasciolopsiasis (giant intestinal fluke) is present in China.

EASTERN SOUTH ASIA includes the countries of Brunei Darussalam, Burma, Democratic Kampuchea, Indonesia, Lao People's Democratic Republic, Malaysia, the Philippines, Singapore, Thailand, and Viet Nam.

Filariasis is present in the rural areas of all of these countries. Malaria is also endemic in rural areas of all these countries except Brunei Darussalam and Singapore. Polio is reported throughout the area, but the incidence is low in Brunei Darussalam and Malaysia, and it has been eliminated in Singapore. Japanese encephalitis and dengue fever occur in epidemics throughout this area. Plague exists in Burma and Viet Nam. Leishmaniasis is present in Burma, and trachoma (an infectious eye disease) is present in Burma, Indonesia, Thailand, and Viet Nam. Mite-borne typhus has been reported in deforested areas.

Food- and water-borne diseases are common. Cholera and other diseases which cause watery diarrhea, amebic and bacillary dysentery, typhoid fever, and viral hepatitis may occur in any of the countries in the area. Schistosomiasis (bilharziasis) is endemic in the Philippines, Indonesia, and the Mekong Delta. Various parasitic diseases such as liver, lung, and intestinal flukes may be acquired throughout the region.

Rabies, snake bites, and leeches are other hazards in this area.

MIDDLE SOUTH ASIA includes Afghanistan, Bangladesh, Bhutan, India, Iran, Maldives, Nepal, Pakistan, and Sri Lanka.

Malaria, leishmaniasis, sandfly fever, brucellosis, hemorrhagic fevers, and polio are risks in this area. Filariasis is common in Bangladesh and India. Leishmaniasis occurs in Afghanistan, India, the Islamic Republic of Iran, and Pakistan. Tick-borne relapsing fever and typhus are reported from Afghanistan, India, and the Islamic Republic of Iran, and typhus occurs in Afghanistan and India. Epidemics of dengue fever may occur in Bangladesh, India, Pakistan, and Sri Lanka, and the hemorrhagic form of the disease has been reported from eastern India and Sri Lanka. Japanese encephalitis has been reported from the eastern part of the area.

Food- and water-borne diseases are common, particularly cholera and other diseases causing watery diarrhea, dysentery, typhoid fever, viral hepatitis, and parasitic worm infections. Giardiasis is common in the Islamic Republic of Iran, and schistosomiasis (bilharziasis) occurs in the southwest part of this country. Trachoma (an infectious eye disease) is common in Afghanistan, India, the Islamic Republic of Iran, Nepal, and Pakistan. Snakes and rabies infection are also hazards in most of these countries.

WESTERN SOUTH ASIA includes what is usually thought of as the Middle East. The countries in this region are: Bahrain, Cyprus, Democratic Yemen, Iraq, Israel, Jordan, Kuwait, Lebanon, Oman, Qatar, Saudi Arabia, Syrian Arab Republic, Turkey, the United Arab Emirates, Yemen.

Malaria exists in certain areas, but not in Kuwait, Bahrain, Cyprus, Israel, Jordan, Lebanon, or Qatar. Some cases of leishmaniasis are reported throughout the area. Murine- and tick-borne typhus can occur in most countries. Tick-borne relapsing fever may occur. A specific type of hemorrhagic fever (Crimean-Congo) has been reported from Iraq. Polio is endemic in this region, but has not been reported from Cyprus in recent years. Trachoma (an infectious eye disease) and rabies may be a problem in many of these countries.

Food-borne and water-borne diseases are a major hazard in this region. Typhoid fever and viral hepatitis exist in all countries, and cholera in many of them. Schistosomiasis (bilharziasis) occurs in Democratic Yemen, Iraq, Saudi Arabia, the Syrian Arab Republic, and Yemen. Parasitic worm infections are also present in many of these countries. Brucellosis is widespread.

Special hazards to pilgrims to Mecca and Medina include heat and water depletion during the hot season.

AFGHANISTAN
Immunization: Y2, H5, T15, Td4, R5
Malaria risk: Throughout country.

BAHRAIN
Immunization: Y2γ, H5, Td5, R5
Malaria risk: None.

BANGLADESH
Immunization: C6, Y2,3, H5, Ra13, Td5, R5, D20
Malaria risk: Throughout country, except no risk in city of Dhaka. Isolated reports of chloroquine resistance.

BHUTAN
Immunization: Y2, H5, T15, Td5, R5
Malaria risk: In rural areas in districts bordering India.

BRUNEI DARUSSALAM
Immunization: Y2γ, H5, Td5, R5, D20
Malaria risk: None.

BURMA
Immunization: Y2,3,7, H5, P10, Ra13, T15, Td5, R5, D20
Malaria risk: In rural areas only. Chloroquine resistance.

CHINA
Immunization: Y2, H4, P10, Td4, R5, D21,24
Malaria risk: In many rural areas. Chloroquine resistance in southern China, including Hainan Island, and areas bordering Lao People's Democratic Republic and Viet Nam.

CYPRUS
Immunization: H4, Td4, R5
Malaria risk: None.

DEMOCRATIC KAMPUCHEA
(formerly Cambodia)
Immunization: Y2, H5, P10, Td5, R5, D20
Malaria risk: Throughout country. Chloroquine resistance.

HONG KONG
Immunization: R5
Malaria risk: None.

INDIA
Immunization: C6,7, Y17,3, H5, P10, Ra13, T15, Td5, R5, D20
Malaria risk: Throughout country. Chloroquine resistance.

INDONESIA
Immunization: C6, Y2,3, H5, Ra13, Td5, R5, D20
Malaria risk: In rural areas, but high risk in all areas of Irian Jaya. No risk in resort areas of Bali. Chloroquine resistance.

IRAN
Immunization: Y2,3γ, H5, P10, T15, Td4, R5
Malaria risk: In rural areas only.

IRAQ
Immunization: Y2, H5, P10, T15, Td5, R5
Malaria risk: In all areas of northern region.

ISRAEL
Immunization: R5
Malaria risk: None.

JAPAN
Immunization: R5
Malaria risk: None.

JORDAN
Immunization: H4, Td4, R5
Malaria risk: None.

KOREA, DEMOCRATIC PEOPLE'S REPUBLIC OF (North)
Immunization: H4, Td4, R5
Malaria risk: None.

KOREA, REPUBLIC OF (South)
Immunization: H4, Td4, R5
Malaria risk: None.

KUWAIT
Immunization: R5
Malaria risk: None.

LAO PEOPLE'S DEMOCRATIC
REPUBLIC
Immunization: Y2, H5, P10, Td5, R5, D20
Malaria risk: Throughout country, except
no risk in city of Vientiane. Chloro-
quine resistance.

LEBANON
Immunization: Y2, R5
Malaria risk: None.

MACAO (Portugal)
Immunization: R5
Malaria risk: None.

MALAYSIA
Immunization: C6, Y2,3γ, H4, Td4, R5,
D20
Malaria risk: In rural areas. Urban and
coastal areas are free from malaria, ex-
cept in Sabah. Chloroquine resistance.

MALDIVES
Immunization: Y2, H5, Td5, R5, D20
Malaria risk: In rural areas, except no risk
in Male Island, Kaafu Atoll, and resort
areas.

MONGOLIA
Immunization: R5
Malaria risk: None.

NEPAL
Immunization: C6, Y2, H5, P10, Ra13,
T15, Td5, R5
Malaria risk: In rural areas in Terai District and Hill Districts below 4,000 feet
(1,200 meters). There is no risk in Kat-
mandu.

OMAN
Immunization: Y2, H5, Td5, R5
Malaria risk: Throughout country.

PAKISTAN
Immunization: C2,6, Y2,3, H5, Ra13,
T15, Td5, R5
Malaria risk: Throughout country. Iso-
lated reports of chloroquine resistance
from the Punjab.

PHILIPPINES
Immunization: C6, Y2γ,19, H4, Ra13,
Td4, R5, D20
Malaria risk: In most rural areas. Some
chloroquine resistance.

QATAR
Immunization: Y2γ, H5, Td5, R5
Malaria risk: None.

SAUDI ARABIA
Immunization: Y2, H5, Td5, R5
Malaria risk: Throughout country, except
no risk in the eastern, northern, and
central provinces, the high altitude areas of Asir Province, and the urban areas of Jeddah, Mecca, Medina, and
Taif.

SINGAPORE
Immunization: Y17γ,3, R5, D20
Malaria risk: None.

SRI LANKA
Immunization: C6, Y2γ, H4, Ra13, Td4,
R5, D20
Malaria risk: Throughout country, except
no risk in Colombo. Isolated reports of
chloroquine resistance.

SYRIAN ARAB REPUBLIC
Immunization: C6, Y2, H5, P10, Td5, R5
Malaria risk: In rural areas only, except
no risk in districts of Deir-es-zor, and
Sweida.

TAIWAN
Immunization: Y2, H4, Td4, R5
Malaria risk: None.

THAILAND
Immunization: C6, Y2γ, H5, Ra13, Td5, R5, D20
Malaria risk: In rural areas. Chloroquine resistance.

TURKEY
Immunization: H4, Ra13, Td4, R5
Malaria risk: In Cukorova/Amikova areas and southeast Anatolia.

UNITED ARAB EMIRATES
Immunization: C6, Y2, H5, Td5, R5
Malaria risk: Throughout country, except no risk in cities of Dubai, Sharjah, Ajman, Umm al Qaiwan, and Emirate of Abu Dhabi.

VIET NAM
Immunization: C6, Y2γ, H4, P10, Ra13, Td4, R5, D20
Malaria risk: In rural areas only, except in the deltas. Chloroquine resistance.

YEMEN ARAB REPUBLIC (Sana'a')
Immunization: Y2γ, H5, Td5, R5
Malaria risk: Throughout country, except no risk in Sada and Haijja provinces.

YEMEN, DEMOCRATIC (Aden)
Immunization: C6, Y2γ, H5, Ra13, Td5, R5
Malaria risk: Throughout country, except no risk in city of Aden or around airport.

EUROPE

NORTHERN EUROPE includes the countries of Belgium, Czechoslovakia, Denmark (with the Faroe Islands), Finland, Federal Republic of Germany, German Democratic Republic, Iceland, Ireland, Luxembourg, Netherlands, Norway, Poland, Sweden, U.S.S.R., United Kingdom (with the Channel Islands and the Isle of Man).

Health hazards to travelers in this area are low, and unlikely to be greater than those found at home, wherever that is. Consequently, the recommended precautions are minimal.

Leishmaniasis exists in this region only in southern U.S.S.R., and tick-borne typhus in east and central Siberia. Tick-borne encephalitis and hemorrhagic fevers may occur in the same areas.

Diarrheal diseases do occur in this region, although the risk is not high in most areas. In the western U.S.S.R., giardiasis is fairly common. Parasitic diseases such as tapeworms are found in parts of northern Europe, especially from freshwater fish around the Baltic Sea area.

Rabies is endemic in animals (especially foxes) in rural areas of this region, except for Iceland, Ireland, the Netherlands, Norway, Sweden, and the United Kingdom.

An environmental health hazard to travelers in northern Europe is the extreme cold in winter.

SOUTHERN EUROPE includes the nations of Albania, Andorra, Austria, Bulgaria, France, Gibraltar, Greece, Hungary, Italy, Liechtenstein, Malta, Monaco, Portugal (with the Azores and Madeira), Romania, San Marino, Spain (with the Canary Islands), Switzerland, Yugoslavia.

Sporadic cases of murine- and tick-borne typhus and mosquito-borne West Nile fever occur in countries bordering the Mediterranean. Leishmaniasis and sandfly fever are also reported from this area. Tick-borne encephalitis and hemorrhagic fevers may occur in the eastern part of this area.

Food- and water-borne diseases include bacillary dysentery and other diarrheas, and typhoid fever, all of which are more common during the summer and autumn, especially in the southeastern and southwestern parts of the area. Brucellosis can occur in the extreme southwest and southeast.

Rabies in animals exists in most of these countries except Gibraltar, Malta, Portugal, and Spain.

ALBANIA
Immunization: C2β, Y2γ, Td4, R5
Malaria risk: None.

ANDORRA
Immunization: R5
Malaria risk: None.

AUSTRIA
Immunization: R5
Malaria risk: None.

BELGIUM
Immunization: R5
Malaria risk: None.

BULGARIA
Immunization: R5
Malaria risk: None.

CZECHOSLOVAKIA
Immunization: R5
Malaria risk: None.

DENMARK (with the Faroe Islands)
Immunization: R5
Malaria risk: None.

FINLAND
Immunization: R5
Malaria risk: None.

FRANCE
Immunization: R5
Malaria risk: None.

GERMAN DEMOCRATIC REPUBLIC
Immunization: R5
Malaria risk: None.

GERMANY, FEDERAL REPUBLIC OF
Immunization: R5
Malaria risk: None.

GIBRALTAR
Immunization: R5
Malaria risk: None.

GREECE
Immunization: Y2β, Td4, R5
Malaria risk: None.

HUNGARY
Immunization: R5
Malaria risk: None.

ICELAND
Immunization: R5
Malaria risk: None.

IRELAND, REPUBLIC OF
Immunization: R5
Malaria risk: None.

ITALY
Immunization: R5
Malaria risk: None.

LIECHTENSTEIN
Immunization: R5
Malaria risk: None.

LUXEMBOURG
Immunization: R5
Malaria risk: None.

MALTA
Immunization: C2, Y2β, R5
Malaria risk: None.

MONACO
Immunization: R5
Malaria risk: None.

NETHERLANDS
Immunization: R5
Malaria risk: None.

NORWAY
Immunization: R5
Malaria risk: None.

POLAND
Immunization: R5
Malaria risk: None.

PORTUGAL (with the Azores and
Madeira)
Immunization: Y2γ,16, R5
Malaria risk: None.

ROMANIA
Immunization: R5
Malaria risk: None.

SAN MARINO
Immunization: R5
Malaria risk: None.

SPAIN (with the Canary Islands)
Immunization: R5
Malaria risk: None.

SWEDEN
Immunization: R5
Malaria risk: None.

SWITZERLAND
Immunization: R5
Malaria risk: None.

U.S.S.R.
Immunization: H4, P10, T15, Td4, R5
Malaria risk: None.

UNITED KINGDOM (with the Channel
Islands and the Isle of Man)
Immunization: R5
Malaria risk: None.

YUGOSLAVIA
Immunization: R5
Malaria risk: None.

OCEANIA (THE SOUTH PACIFIC)

In AUSTRALIA and NEW ZEALAND the risk of acquiring a communicable disease is low, and considered to be no greater than that found in the traveler's own country, no matter where that is.

Mosquito-borne diseases such as viral encephalitis may occur in some rural areas of Australia. Dengue fever is present in parts of Northern Queensland and the Torres Strait islands. Among diseases contracted through contaminated food and water, meningoencephalitis has been reported.

Other miscellaneous risks include the hazard to swimmers from coral and jellyfish, and the effects of extreme heat in the northern and central parts of Australia.

MELANESIA and MICRONESIA-POLYNESIA includes the islands of American Samoa, Cook Islands, Fiji, French Polynesia (Tahiti), Guam, Kiribati, Nauru, New Caledonia, Niue, Papua New Guinea, Samoa, Solomon Islands, Tonga, Trust Territory of the Pacific Islands, Tuvalu, Vanuatu.

Malaria is endemic in Papua New Guinea, and is found as far east and south as Vanuatu. Mite-borne typhus and polio are also present in Papua New Guinea. Trachoma (an infectious eye disease) occurs in parts of Melanesia. Filariasis is widespread in the entire region. Dengue fever, including its hemorrhagic form, can occur in epidemics on most of the islands. Japanese encephalitis has been reported.

Food-borne and water-borne diseases such as diarrheal illness, typhoid fever, and parasitic worm infections are common. Illness may occur from eating raw or cooked fish or shellfish.

Other risks include such hazards to swimmers as coral, poisonous fish, and sea snakes.

AMERICAN SAMOA
Immunization: Y2γ, R5, D21
Malaria risk: None.

AUSTRALIA
Immunization: Y2,3γ, H4, R5, D20,22
Malaria risk: None.

COOK ISLANDS (New Zealand)
Immunization: R5, D21
Malaria risk: None.

FIJI
Immunization: Y2γ, R5, D21
Malaria risk: None.

FRENCH POLYNESIA (including Tahiti)
Immunization: Y2γ, R5, D20
Malaria risk: None.

GUAM
Immunization: R5
Malaria risk: None.

KIRIBATI (formerly Gilbert Islands)
Immunization: Y2γ, H5, Td5, R5
Malaria risk: None.

NAURU ISLAND
Immunization: Y2γ, R5, D21
Malaria risk: None.

NEW CALEDONIA (France)
Immunization: Y2,3β, H5, Td5, R5, D20
Malaria risk: None.

NEW ZEALAND
Immunization: R5
Malaria risk: None.

NIUE ISLAND (New Zealand)
Immunization: Y2γ, R5, D21
Malaria risk: None.

PACIFIC ISLANDS, TRUST
TERRITORY OF THE U.S.A.
Immunization: R5, D21
Malaria risk: None.

PAPUA NEW GUINEA
Immunization: Y2γ, H5, Td5, R5, D20
Malaria risk: Throughout country.
   Chloroquine resistance.

SAMOA (formerly Western Samoa)
Immunization: Y2γ, R5, D21
Malaria risk: None.

SAMOA, AMERICAN (see American
Samoa)

SOLOMON ISLANDS
Immunization: Y2, R5, D20
Malaria risk: Throughout country.
   Chloroquine resistance.

TAHITI (see French Polynesia)

TONGA
Immunization: Y2γ, R5, D21
Malaria risk: None.

TUVALU (formerly Ellice Islands)
Immunization: Y2γ, R5
Malaria risk: None.

VANUATU (formerly New Hebrides)
Immunization: H5, Td5, R5, D20
Malaria risk: Throughout country, except
   no risk on Fortuna Island.

INDEX